Finding Health After Cancer

Stories of Renewal and Healing

by Deb Nelson

Stay curious.
Keep asking
questions!
Deb Nelson

Published by deb nelson consulting, llc.
P.O. Box 234
Yarmouth, ME 04096

www.bewellcg.com

Editor: Kate Victory Hannisian, Blue Pencil Consulting
Book and Cover Design: Grace Peirce, Great Life Press
greatlifepress.com

Print ISBN: 978-0-9988894-0-5
Ebook ISBN: 978-0-9988894-1-2
Library of Congress Control Number: 2018948101

Disclaimer:
This book is written as a source of information only. The author is not a doctor and has no medical training. The information contained in this book should by no means be considered a substitute for the advice of a qualified medical professional, who should always be consulted before beginning any health program. The reader is cautioned to carefully assess the risks associated with following any health program and is responsible for obtaining health care appropriate for his/her condition.

Photo credits:
Front Cover: Rows 1 and 2 Photos by Richard Sawyer Photography; Row 3 (l to r) Photos by Jaclyn Rae Photography, Pyxie Studios, Bret Reynoso
Back Cover: Photo by Richard Sawyer Photography

Praise for Finding Health After Cancer: Stories of Renewal and Healing

When I was initially diagnosed, I knew very little about cancer, treatments or choices. I made medical decisions based on the severity of my circumstances. However, once treatment was complete, I immediately sought out alternative paths to improve my health and embrace the journey of survival. I would have loved to have this book to connect with other individual survival stories and tap into available resources and options.

Yvonne Devine, 17-year survivor

In *Finding Health After Cancer: Stories of Renewal and Healing*, Deb Nelson has pulled together a wonderful collection of stories that illustrate just how personal and varied the path to healing can be. This book serves as a reminder that, even when facing a diagnosis as frightening as cancer, it is critical to look at all your options and choose the path to health that is right for you. These stories provide not only inspiration and hope but also serve as a great resource for all cancer patients seeking to find their own road.

I look forward to recommending this book to all my cancer patients.

Graham Haynes, MAOM, LAc
Whole Health Acupuncture and Herbal Medicine
Yarmouth, ME
www.acupunctureinmaine.com

The quality of your life is determined by the quality of the questions you ask. The cancer survivors in this book were asked, "What was the most important question you asked following your cancer diagnosis?" The answer to this question, though different for each survivor, determined the quality of their life. They asked important questions, got relevant answers and acted upon those answers. After twenty-one years of being a chiropractor, I have seen paths to health look different for different people. There are many right answers to "What was the most important question you asked?" This book highlights how those questions and answers lead to not only surviving, but thriving.

Dr. Christine E. Maguire
Family Chiropractic Associates
Scarborough, ME
scarboroughfamilychiro.com

There are many ways people can heal, live and survive cancer. The personal and very different narratives of hope in *Finding Health After Cancer* . . . expresses the different healing paths taken when people face, address and walk through their process towards renewal. Traditional, complementary, alternative and integrative approaches to health and healing are respectfully reflected here. Enriching and empowering, I feel just hearing these stories can be healing, too. Perhaps they may help to reduce feelings of isolation and loneliness, which can come along with a diagnosis. They may help to open us up to what's possible through witnessing how unique each person's healing journey can be.

Lucrezia Mangione, NCC, LCPC, DCEP, CMT, CHTP/I
Handcrafted Health
Silver Spring, MD
www.handcrafted-health.com

Never before have we had access to such incredible amounts of information and been able to regularly tap into expert opinion. Yet in the management of our own health, or when faced with a cancer diagnosis, it always comes down to the question of finding that "best" choice for treatment. The diverse stories in Deb's book are a testament to the complexity of that choice and the importance of individualized care. It is also an enlightening illustration of the part of the process that can be more terrifying than researching treatment options: designing a healing journey for you, and you alone. Hearing these personal stories of treatment and lifestyle evolution is the necessary precursor to empowerment and self-advocacy. I look forward to sharing these accounts with my own patients and I thank Deb for bringing these stories to light.

Aline R. Potvin, ND
Your Own Wellness
Biddeford, ME
www.arpnaturod.com

Photo credits

Contents

Dedication

It is with great honor and respect that I dedicate this book to the memory of Tim Hussey. I learned that Tim had been diagnosed with mucosal melanoma when a friend emailed me a link to his blog, *Beating It: Tim's Journey in Kicking Cancer in the Ass.* Tim began writing his blog in August 2014, three months after his diagnosis, and continued to post several times a month until May 2016. Here, Tim shared the insights he gained while undergoing treatment: his thoughts, fears, hopes, and experiences. Those of us who read his blog got a glimpse into the inner workings of Tim's brilliant mind. His thoughts were with his family, friends, and colleagues as he shared the highs and lows, seemingly without much of a filter, of his life-changing diagnosis.

In a blog post on October 28, 2014, Tim reflected on a commencement speech he gave at York County Community College just thirteen days before being diagnosed with cancer. He asked the graduating students to consider how they would fill their dash: how would they fill that space between birth and death? To guide them in answering that question, Tim encouraged the graduates to complete what he called an Ethical Will. Joking that no lawyers are needed to complete this document, Tim explained that:

> *An Ethical Will is a special place where you get to document your core values and your life lessons, that you want to leave to your loved ones and your friends. It's not about your hard assets or your estate. It's about what REALLY matters. Your true legacy, the one that matters most, is how you live your life and what choices you make. Documenting this in an ethical will can be a very powerful moment in*

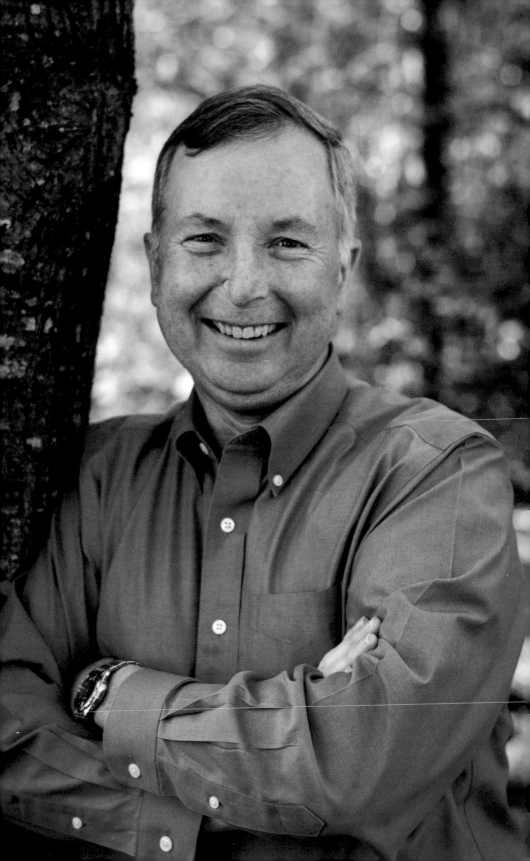

your life. You declare to yourself what really matters, and you ultimately leave these lessons to your loved ones. This is how legacy is truly created in a purposeful way.

And that is how Tim Hussey lived—he kept his core values front and center every day of his life. When his cancer returned, Tim continued to lead his life following those values. He worked from home, received visitors at his home, and focused on his family. Because while many people enjoyed being in the company of Tim Hussey, everyone knew that Tim's family came first—always.

Tim's legacy is based on his values—compassion, personal integrity, and commitment to community—values that made him a well-respected and beloved leader of his family's company, of his local community, and the larger state community. This legacy will touch future generations because Tim had the forethought to establish The Timothy B. Hussey Leadership Fund. This fund will create a leadership program that builds Maine's future leaders while addressing Tim's wish to continue the legacy of his family by supporting innovation, entrepreneurship, and perseverance.

Tim's family has launched a website where you can read Tim's story, and learn more about and contribute to The Timothy B. Hussey Leadership Fund: www.timhusseyleadershipfund.org

Tim taught many of us about life, leadership, and community prior to his cancer diagnosis. What he continued to teach us after his cancer diagnosis, and through the last days of his life, is equally powerful. Upon learning his mass was malignant, Tim recalled saying to his doctor: "Well, we don't get to choose the hand we are dealt in life, we only get to choose how we play the cards." Well played, Tim, well played.

Gratitude

Writing this book has taken me down a path I never pictured in my wildest dreams. I've had the opportunity to talk with and learn from amazing people—cancer survivors, caregivers, activists, medical personnel, and more. My deepest thanks to each person who took the time to talk with me, listen to me, and share their stories—whether publicly or privately.

Thank you to all the people who host conferences and provide a forum for cancer patients, caregivers, and advocates to gather and learn from one another. Whether online or in person, these conferences confirm for each of us that we are not alone as we seek answers to the questions we hoped we'd never have to ask.

Thank you to each person who was brave enough to include their stories in this book. Each of these people made a conscious decision to share their experience in finding a path to health with me, and then with all of you who are now reading this book. I am so grateful they trusted me to help tell those stories.

Many thanks to Maura Halkiotis, who introduced me to the world of activism for cancer patients through fundraising and was also kind enough to share her story in this book. Ray Inglesi taught me the importance of listening to my inner voice and encouraged me to walk through those open doors I was facing. Michelle Neujahr provided encouragement, structure, and accountability as I explored the world of writing and publishing this book.

Deborah McLean, Sande Updegraph, and Kym Dakin-Neal have been my sisters in accountability, supporting me as I put the pieces of this book and my business together. And then there's my editor, Kate Victory Hannisian, who stood by me with her amazing combination of patience and persistence as I pushed and missed deadlines. As a first-time author, I relied heavily on Kate's expertise—and did I mention her patience?

Thanks to Grace Peirce for the design and layout of this book and for sharing her knowledge and expertise as she guided me through the logistics involved with getting this book printed and available to readers.

Thank you to each of the photographers who provided the photos for this book. The power of these photos is evident to me, as each image captures the essence of each person and their story. Special thanks to Dick Sawyer for coordinating with photographers around the country and for his guidance to me at every step in publishing this book. You'll notice that Dick took many of the photos that appear in the book; his expertise, flexibility, and sense of humor were key in getting this book to print.

And, of course, thank you to my husband, John, for believing in me, cheering me on, and supporting me as I navigated the publishing world. Each and every day, John is in my corner as I never imagined someone could be. Each and every day, John is by my side. Each and every day, John encourages me to be me. For this and so much more, I am grateful beyond words.

Foreword

Stories help us make sense of our lives. This project offers hope for those who are newly diagnosed with cancer and looking for resources. But just as importantly, this book is an opportunity for the featured cancer survivors to reflect upon and give meaning to their own cancer stories. As a primary care physician, I have learned that the most important part of my job is drawing a *story* out of the patient as I take their medical *history*. While the details may appear irrelevant to the diagnosis through the lens of our Western medicine model, allowing the patient time and space to contemplate their lives in the context of their health can be more healing for them than anything else I could offer. Stories create an underlying sense of intention—they shift the power to the patient, the central character, who has the ability to act rather than only be acted upon. Making sense of our stories—the stories of our bodies, our minds, and our spirits—is an essential step in creating wholeness. My job is to support patients to re-imagine themselves as creators, rather than victims, of those narratives.

As an MD trained in integrative medicine, I appreciate how Deb Nelson's unbiased approach recognizes that there are many different paths to health and she does not proselytize any particular healing system. In my mind, any kind of meaningful "complementary and alternative" approach to cancer treatment attempts to give agency back to the protagonist of the story. Whether that is by diet, detoxification, stress management, spirituality, exercise, or supplements, the goal is to lay down the healthiest possible foundation in order to give your immune system the greatest chance of overcoming the cancer cells. "Conventional" medicine may be miraculous, but it is not perfect. Our coming of age in medicine occurred in concert with the birth of machines and the industrial revolution. The human body was seen as a machine—with different parts working in unison to create a whole, functioning person. If one part broke, you replaced it. We have become experts in ever-more microscopic parts of the machine. But has this come at the sacrifice of the whole? Dutch anthropologist Louis Bolk said it eloquently: "We are in the habit of investigating life through magnifying glasses, of thus bringing otherwise invisible matter within our field of vision; how different, how much larger our concept of life would be if it were possible to study through minimizing glasses and thus bring within our field of vision matters that are beyond the reach of the eye, taking as a goal of our studies the cohesion of the phenomena, rather than the analysis of matter?" Have we become so obsessed with details that we have forgotten the whole? In essence, is this "disintegration" detrimental to our health?

Healing from cancer should be a story of unification rather than separation, wholeness rather than "disintegration." Stories help us create coherence out of what might seem like discrete parts. I don't like it when there are three parties in the ring: the cancer, the oncologist, and the "alternative." As an "integrative" provider, I try to unify the team. Let's use the best of all modalities, conventional and "everything else," to help patients heal within the context of their own lives. In other words, we widen our toolbox, becoming more open, rather than narrow. In Bolk's sense, we use our "minimizing glasses" to see the larger story. This may mean pharmaceuticals and this may mean meditation. It may mean surgery and it may mean energy healing. It may mean reflection upon how this diagnosis fits into the larger picture, the whole story. I am a strong believer that the intention with which we enter any treatment plan plays a large part in the outcome. Healing has to occur in the context of our own stories. There is never a one-size-fits-all approach to health; that completely undermines the story of the individual patient sitting in front of me.

Often stuck in the middle of conventional and nonconventional philosophies about cancer and healing, I am deeply inspired by the stories Deb shares. Each person figured out how to integrate the best tools at their disposal to create health. All the journeys are unique, but underlying them all is a theme of openness, exploration, and reflection. Their stories changed when cancer entered their lives, but cancer itself propelled these survivors on a new path toward self-efficacy and advocacy.

Elizabeth Strawbridge, MD
Portland, ME

Introduction

Almost every time I tell someone that I'm writing a book that shares the stories of people who found health after cancer, there's a pause in the conversation. Then the person might shift in her chair and ask me if I'm writing this book because of my own cancer diagnosis. No, I've never had a cancer diagnosis. So what the heck am I doing writing this book?

Here's the short story: While training for a triathlon to raise funds in support of cancer patients and their families living in Maine, I read Brendan Brazier's book *Thrive: The Vegan Nutrition Guide to Optimal Performance in Sports and Life.* One simple phrase in that book spurred me on to ask questions, which in turn, has taken me on a journey I could never have imagined: "It is impossible for cancer to develop in an alkaline environment." There was no footnote to provide information validating that statement. There was no qualifier indicating some people believe this to be true, or that some studies indicate this to be the case. It was a statement of fact similar to 1 + 1 = 2. That was the first time I had seen or heard the phrase "alkaline environment." So, I folded the page over. When I finished reading the book, I returned to the page I had folded over and started walking down a path that would change my life.

I started reading every book I could get my hands on to learn about the relationship between cancer and an alkaline diet—and, believe me, there is no shortage of books on this topic! I talked with cancer survivors who graciously shared their stories with me. I researched the history of alkalinity online. I attended conferences to learn about cancer treatment—the history, current practices, and plans for the future.

What I learned from studying brave cancer conquerors is that there are many paths to health. Each person you'll read about in this book faced a life-challenging and life-changing moment in his or her own way. Each of these cancer conquerors was forced to make a variety of decisions as they navigated their path to health. Priorities shifted without warning as they learned their diagnosis. They began asking questions, listening to friends and family members, tuning in to their intuition, and researching options.

The stories share the information I learned. Each person you'll meet in this book transformed his or her life following a cancer diagnosis. Treatment varied from person to person: some people followed a conventional treatment plan, while others turned to complementary and alternative treatment.

I was shocked to learn that there were so many paths to health and that lifestyle choices can impact our health even more than genetics. That is *why* I've written this book: I was also struck by the fact that I had gathered information that isn't readily available to all cancer patients. If any of my friends or family members were diagnosed with cancer, I'd want them to know that they had choices to make surrounding their treatment—that they *could* and *should* take an active role in their treatment plan.

With cancer diagnoses being estimated for one in two men and one in three women, it's likely each one of us will be affected at least indirectly by cancer in our lifetime. As environmental factors continue to change and influence our health, we all have the opportunity to direct the course of our health. Hearing the words "You have cancer" can easily send people into a tailspin. The people you'll meet in this book found a way to steer clear of a downward spiral. They looked at their options, decided which treatment suited their particular situation, and forged ahead. They also became advocates for themselves and other cancer patients.

Should you or a loved one be faced with a cancer diagnosis, I hope these stories provide inspiration to you as you identify your path to health.

Note to readers: *Many, if not all, of the people who are sharing their stories in this book could appear in more than one chapter. I've chosen to include each of them in the chapter that illustrates key elements of their path to health.*

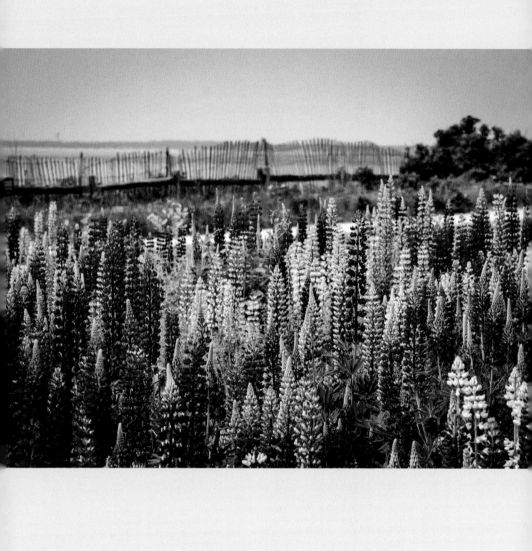

Living the Good Life After Conventional Treatment

T HE FIVE PEOPLE highlighted in this chapter chose surgery, chemotherapy, and radiation—or some combination thereof—to treat their cancer. They asked lots of questions along the way as they weighed the options presented to them, conducted their own research, and sought advice from friends and family prior to undergoing treatment.

Each person had a different set of personal circumstances to weigh as they identified the course of treatment they would follow. What they have in common is a humbleness and a willingness to become advocates for others in their community.

As a medical doctor, **Anne Brown** is in a unique position to walk beside and guide her patients on their path to health. Anne's personal experience in cancer treatment inspired her to enroll in a Fellowship in Integrative Medicine. Her focus is now on the mind-body connection, a significant adjustment to her professional life following her cancer diagnosis.

Focusing on health had always been important for **John Curtin**. Following a cancer diagnosis, he continued both his exercise and supplement routine. He also shares his experience—that this combination of exercise and nutrition regimen is what helped him recover so quickly—with people through his work.

Maura Halkiotis is well-known in her community through her visible professional and volunteer work. She's become a valuable resource for anyone in her small seacoast town who has a cancer diagnosis. Following her treatment, Maura made exercise and plant-based food key elements of her lifestyle. She raised funds to support those who were going through treatment as well as to support research efforts to treat cancer.

Bob Johnson has also become a resource for his community. Whether it's to raise funds to support programs at a local cancer center or to speak at a conference about growing a business, Bob is the first to step in to lend a hand. Following his diagnosis Bob left his job, which was a pretty big deal, as he was cofounder of the company. Then he moved from Vermont to Maine where he, along with two colleagues, started a "small neighborhood artisan bakery that wakes up early every day to bring you our special brand of small batch lovin' from the oven." What a lucky neighborhood!

Carroll Tiernan turned to nature when cancer arrived at her doorstep. No surprise here, since Carroll worked for years at Maine Audubon. A force to be reckoned with herself, Carroll found that yoga calmed and grounded her as she went through her treatment.

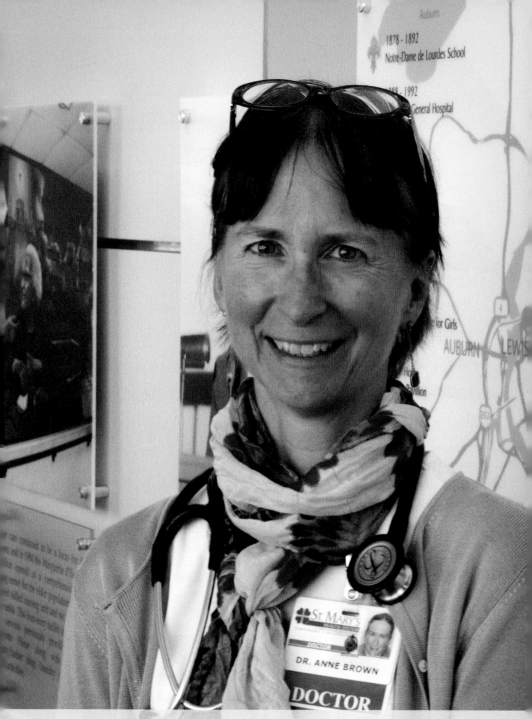

"Trust your instinct. It usually comes from deep inside—a place that is often more tuned in to the body than our thinking mind."

ANNE BROWN, MD

Diagnosis: Stage IIIa breast cancer
Treatment: Chemotherapy, surgery, radiation

How did you change your diet and/or lifestyle following your cancer diagnosis? At whose suggestion?

I changed diet and lifestyle gradually and dramatically after my diagnosis. No one suggested that I do this. I was told "eat healthy and exercise." I believed before (and still do) that cancer is a "multi-hit" disease. This means that multiple factors have to be in place or out of place to result in the body having the correct milieu for cancer to grow and then for the gene that triggers it to be "hit" by something (i.e., a virus or toxin) and the immune system is not at its peak performance to correct this process.

There were two major reasons for my change. First, during my treatment I thought a lot and read a lot about diet and lifestyle. Second, I read *Healing and the Mind* by Bill Moyers, which was life-altering. Many of the experts interviewed for that book felt there was an emotional trauma or stress connection with breast cancer.

I evaluated my diet/lifestyle very honestly and found that there were several things that I was not doing well at all. I looked at four areas of my life: diet/nutrition, activity/exercise, relaxation/mind-body, and environment. For diet/nutrition, there is a tremendous amount of information and misinformation available. (I feel like I am still learning.) Along with my treatment,

I was given a handout that was useless. I went to see an oncology dietician. This was helpful for learning about the American Institute for Cancer Research (AICR). This organization is a reputable source of large studies on the basics for nutrition. Based on this, I increased my consumption of fruits and vegetables from four to five total servings a day to five vegetables and three fruits a day, cut way back on saturated/total fats, added some whole grains, stopped eating any foods with nitrates, and decided to avoid all alcohol. This consult was not enough. After starting my fellowship in integrative medicine and meeting health coach Kendall Scott, I learned much more about macro/micronutrients. I added daily cruciferous vegetables, cut way back on foods with a high glycemic index, increased healthy fats, increased whole grains to three to five a day, and started looking at organic foods. I am still learning.

With regard to exercise, I read studies that indicated thirty minutes of moderate exercise five days a week is the bare minimum, and that having more vigorous exercise, and more time than 200 minutes a week, has added benefit. I really was only walking four to five miles a week and occasionally playing tennis. Now I try very hard to walk/run fifteen miles a week. I reach this goal 90% of the time. In the winter, I do an exercise bike and snowshoeing as well. I found that I was very weak after all my treatments and seem to be really predisposed to muscle, tendon, and ligament injury, so I am trying to stretch more and plan to add strength training to my routine.

My biggest area of need was in relaxation/mind-body medicine. I have done extensive reading, research, and training in this area as a result of my cancer diagnosis. I meditate daily, aiming for thirty to forty minutes a day. It was hard to do at first, but is great now that I have made it a habit. I am practicing mindfulness on a regular basis and still trying to increase this and learn more about it. I have made a commitment to sleeping at least seven and a half to eight hours a night and to taking more time and giving myself permission to have fun or do something for myself. This has resulted in stepping away from a busy primary care practice that included on-call, hospital, and office work. This was very hard to do and I still feel a little guilt over this decision.

After attending a conference and a training session in mind-body medicine, I went on to enroll in a fellowship in integrative medicine. The fellowship has been transformative personally and professionally. I see mind-body medicine and integrative medicine as my new career. In my primary care practice, I was disillusioned with the lack of time I could spend discussing health and wellness and the lack of expertise that I had—my only solutions were often pharmaceuticals. There is a definite place for pharmaceuticals—I would not be alive today had I not had chemotherapy—but it is for treatment of active, significant disease, not for prevention and common day-to-day ailments.

Finally, I think the environment that I live in is important and I am starting to research and think about this and make changes such as eating organic foods, avoiding processed foods, avoiding BPA in plastics/cans, and starting to get away from a lot of chemicals in household cleaning and toiletries.

What treatment/lifestyle modification do you feel worked best for you? And why?

I believe that all the things I have done have made my body/internal milieu a much healthier place for my immune system to function in and cancer less likely to grow in. Avoiding toxins is important. I think the diet change made a very big difference as it had been at least 50% toxic, even though I thought I was not doing bad. When I recorded it regularly and really looked at it, my diet was not great. I feel healthier since eating better and feel like my immune system is stronger.

The physical exercise is great for stress reduction and also for making me stronger, not to mention that it feels fantastic to do it and that feeling lasts for several hours after. There is a lot of new research showing how key exercise is. I think the mind-body work/mindfulness is the most important so far, since I have always internalized and suppressed stress and there seems to be a strong connection between breast cancer and emotional stress.

What treatment(s) do you continue to follow?

I am done with my medical/pharmaceutical treatments. I see my diet, exercise, and meditation as a form of preventative treatment.

What do you wish you had known when you were diagnosed? What advice do you have for someone receiving a cancer diagnosis today?

I wish I had known about integrative medicine and had the option to have a consult with an integrative medicine physician looking specifically at oncology. I also wish I had access to a mind-body group to participate in and guide my learning in mind-body techniques as I was finishing treatment. It would have helped a lot.

What did you learn from having cancer?

I have learned how precious each and every day is. I really understand how uncertain the future is and therefore I try very hard not to "put things off." I love living in the moment and find it so rewarding, especially being around my kids and family. I have learned that I should be living my priorities first and not have them just be intentions. I have adjusted my life dramatically to spend more time with my family, more time taking care of them and myself, and I have changed my work to a career where I can be more helpful to people who have a cancer diagnosis or who just want to be healthier.

What else would you like to share?

I want to thank my family and friends who helped me through this difficult time and thank my mentors, classmates, and peers who have helped and guided me in starting the oncology mind-body program at St. Mary's. I also am really excited to complete my integrative medicine fellowship and be able to bring this specialty to St. Mary's (where I work) and to the greater Lewiston-Auburn (Maine) community.

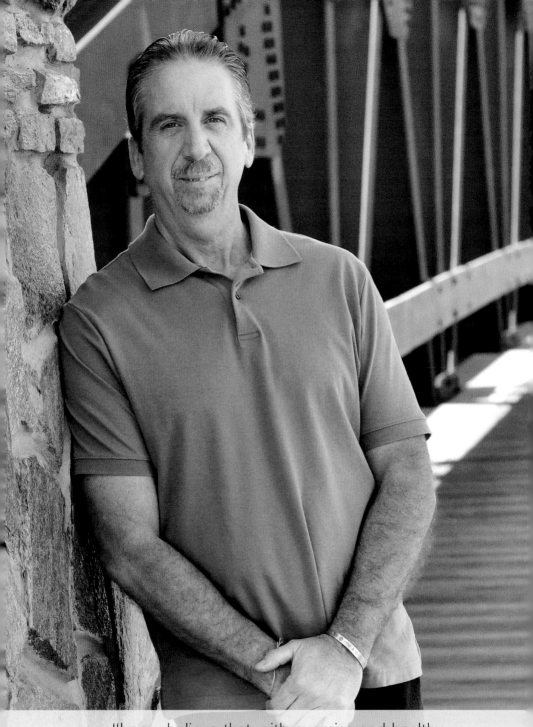

"I now believe that with exercise and healthy eating you can lick cancer. Stay positive and find people who will be there for you no matter what!"

JOHN CURTIN

Diagnosis: Stage IV squamous cell tongue cancer
Treatment: Chemotherapy and radiation

What was the most important question you asked following your cancer diagnosis?

Actually, there were two:

> *What is the survival rate?*
> *What is my life expectancy?*

How did you change your diet and/or lifestyle following your cancer diagnosis?

I did a lot of research and followed some suggestions in the book *Killing Cancer–Not People*—particularly when it came to dietary changes. I eliminated red meats, processed food and sugar, most dairy, alcohol, and other food products that lent themselves to keeping my body acidic. I also added more vegetables, fruits, chicken, and salmon to my diet.

Since I was always in good shape, going to the gym four to five times a week, there was no change to my exercise routine. And no, I never smoked or chewed tobacco, go figure! This wasn't a change, but I've been taking Reliv nutritional products and truly believe that my recovery was so much quicker because of them. And the doctors were amazed at how quickly I was able to have my feeding tube removed and get back to the gym.

What treatment/lifestyle modification do you feel worked best for you? And why?

Exercise is a great way to keep the pounds off, reduce stress, and feel better. The news continues to come in about processed food and sugar and it's all bad. So I truly believe that staying away from these foods has helped with me feeling good. And continuing the Reliv products.

What did you learn from having cancer?

Try to live life to the fullest. I was healthy prior to the diagnosis and this hit me from left field, so you never know.

What else would you like to share?

I can't stress enough the importance of doing your own research. There are many so-called remedies that are really "out there," and I always adhere to the KIS (keep it simple) method. Exercise and healthy nutrition!

John continues to work at Wealth Thru Nutrition—"The Nutritional Epigenetics Company" (www.WealthThruNutrition.com).

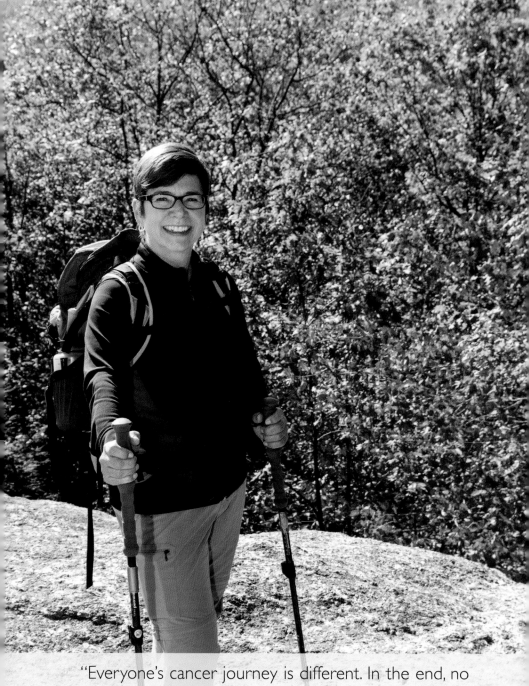

"Everyone's cancer journey is different. In the end, no matter the outcome, you need to be able to accept that the decisions you made were the best ones you could make for yourself."

Diagnosis: Stage IIa breast cancer
Treatment: Mastectomy and reconstruction, chemotherapy, five years of Tamoxifen, five years of Femara

What was the most important question you asked following your cancer diagnosis?

Can I get a second opinion in Boston?

How did you change your diet and/or lifestyle following your cancer diagnosis? At whose suggestion?

In the year prior to my diagnosis I had lost about thirty pounds through diet and exercise. After my treatments, I put the weight back on, about thirteen pounds the first year, then twenty in the second year. My diet and exercise regime fluctuated over the next eight years with little or no results until 2008, when I had an awakening. Two things happened that year. First, I somehow got talked into signing up for a duathlon as part of an all-women's sporting event to raise money for the Maine Cancer Foundation. The funny thing was I didn't run and I certainly didn't ride a bike—I didn't even own one. Second, I saw the movie *Eating*, which is about the link between diet and disease.

In that year, I started exercising—running, biking and strength training—and switched to a vegetarian diet. Over the next two years I lost thirty pounds. In 2009 I added swimming and competed in a full sprint triathlon. Since then I have competed in a number of 5K and 10K races, two half-marathons, seven sprint triathlons and a number of fifty-plus-mile bike rides. I also love to hike and have summited both Mount Katahdin (Maine) and Mount Washington (New Hampshire).

What treatment/lifestyle modification do you feel worked best for you? And why?

I don't think I'd be alive today if I hadn't had the initial mastectomy and chemotherapy, but I owe my long-term health to the lifestyle changes I began in 2008 (both diet and exercise).

What do you wish you had known when you were diagnosed? What advice do you have for someone receiving a cancer diagnosis today?

Although there is a lot more information out there today than in 1999, I feel pretty confident that I had adequate information to make the choices I did. Initially I was going to have a different treatment (partial mastectomy, radiation and chemotherapy) in Maine, but when I went to Boston for my second opinion they proposed a different route. Although it was more radical, I believe it saved my life.

For anyone diagnosed with cancer today I would say this: Do your homework, talk to more than one doctor, ask questions and be prepared to make your own decisions. Also, have a "buddy." Someone who will go to the doctor with you to take notes. Someone who will push you. Someone who will ask questions you might not be willing to ask.

What did you learn from having cancer?

I learned to live! I love my life and I owe that to my cancer diagnosis. It made me think differently at every decision point in my life. It made me brave. It gave me confidence. It reminded me of the things I loved as a young woman and brought those back to me. It made me less tolerant of people who wanted to bring me down. I have made friends and lost friends because of cancer. I realize that life is too short to be dragged down by people who don't share my love for life. I can still love them, but from afar.

What else would you like to share?

I still don't know why some people die of cancer and others don't. Some people believe in traditional medicine. Others believe in healing their bodies naturally. No matter what course a person takes, I do believe in the words of oncologist O. Carl Simonton: "In the face of uncertainty, there is nothing wrong with hope."

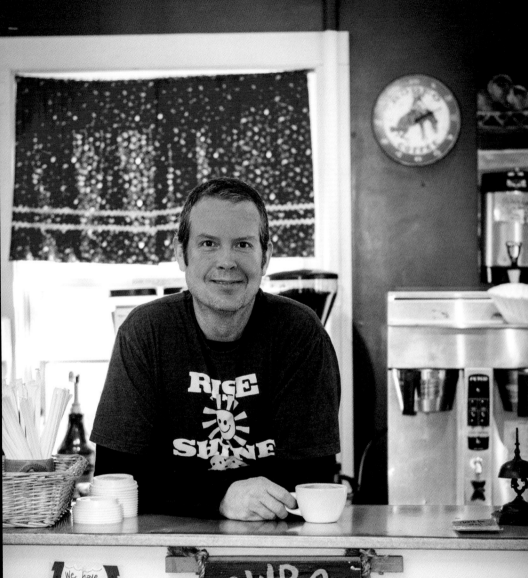

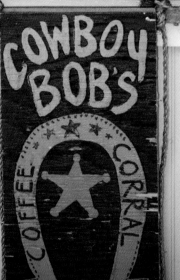

Diagnosis: Stage I testicular cancer

Treatment: Surgery, chemo. When he was diagnosed at age thirty-seven in 2007, Bob followed conventional treatment for his cancer and then took a look at where his life was heading.

What was the most important question you asked following your cancer diagnosis?

What's my prognosis?

How did you change your diet and/or lifestyle following your cancer diagnosis?

My diet stayed the same before, during and after my treatment. The changes I made focused on my lifestyle: curbing and managing stress.

I decided that I didn't have the drive to stay at my job—as the owner/cofounder of a fast-growth company, I began to feel the need to recalibrate my time. I wanted to be involved with a smaller company, so I left my job.

I took some time to think about what kind of life I wanted to have. I moved to Maine and started a new company, Scratch Baking Co.

What treatment do you continue to follow?

Annual CT scans, chest X-rays, blood work.

What treatment/lifestyle modification do you feel worked best for you? And why?

My eyes are open to experiencing all that life has to offer. I've come to recognize that the bus is rolling down the street really fast—if you're not looking, it can sneak up on you. Be awake in life.

What advice do you have for someone receiving a cancer diagnosis today?

Manage your care:

Take charge of your treatment.

Make sure your questions get answered.

Remember that the medical community works for you.

What did you learn from having cancer?

I learned to find balance in work and play, and to appreciate every day.

Bob is the cofounder of Scratch Baking Co., and was cofounder of Magic Hat Brewing Co. when he was diagnosed.

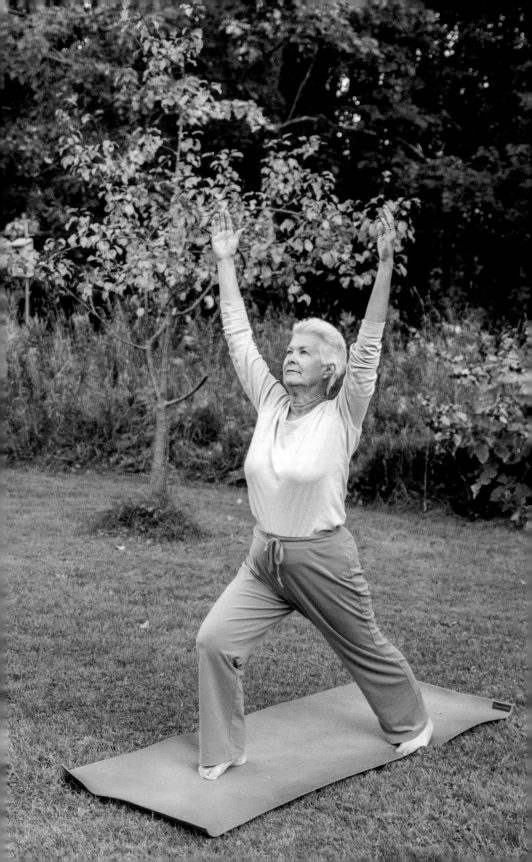

Diagnosis: Stage IV ovarian cancer
Treatment: Chemo, surgery, four more rounds of chemo. Diagnosed at age seventy in 2013, Carroll discovered the healing power of yoga following surgery and chemo.

What was the most important question you asked following your cancer diagnosis?

What do we do now?

How did you change your diet and/or lifestyle following your cancer diagnosis?

I stopped putting off those small pleasures in life.

I felt that moving lymph was important and talked with three yoga teachers to help me develop a daily practice using these asanas. I follow this practice religiously every day.

What treatment/lifestyle modification do you feel worked best for you? And why?

Yoga was the most important addition to getting all signs of cancer out of my lymph nodes. Otherwise, I listened very closely to my body and what it seemed to need.

"Use the good china, i.e. now is the time to enjoy, not later."

What advice do you have for someone receiving a cancer diagnosis today?

First, take a deep breath. It is not fun, but it is doable. Stay away from the web; there is too much negative, worst-case information. Do what feels right to you.

What else would you like to share?

It was an amazing learning experience. It opened my heart in a new way to receiving from friends and well-wishers. There are many, many wonderful people willing to help.

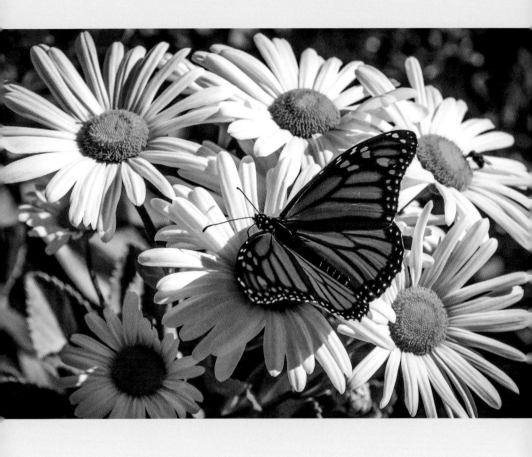

— 2 —

Plan B: When Surgery, Chemo, and Radiation Aren't the Answer

WITH HIGH HOPES for conventional treatment healing their cancer, the three people sharing their stories in this chapter realized Plan A was not working for them. After completing treatment, they either had a recurrence or were told there was nothing more that could be done for them. Not satisfied with the options offered to them and not ready to succumb, these cancer conquerors forged their own paths to health.

Stuart Cobb was diagnosed with brain cancer and underwent surgery and chemotherapy. After being told he was cancer-free, he and his wife, Kristen, celebrated their good fortune. Their celebration was short-lived, however, when they learned six months later that the cancer had returned. The treatment plan their doctor suggested was chemo. Stuart endured one more treatment and told his wife he'd rather die than continue the treatment. Kristen began researching alternative treatment options that proved successful for

Stuart. They credit their faith and alternative therapies for Stuart's health today. The Cobbs have become advocates for brain cancer patients, speaking publicly to warn of the dangers of cell phone use and the connection to brain cancer.

After **Joyce Foley** was diagnosed with ovarian cancer, her treatment plan included surgery and chemotherapy. Not wanting to draw attention to herself, Joyce also chose not to go public with her diagnosis. She changed her mind during her treatment, realizing that the support of friends and family was critical to her healing. She had the support of Sister Gladys and all of the nuns in her convent, all pulling for Joyce and saying prayers for her health. This was a boost to Joyce, as she had two recurrences. After the second recurrence, Joyce chose not have any more chemo. Instead, she adopted a plant-based diet and added herbal supplements to her regimen.

Joyce also began a program to give other cancer patients a boost during their treatment. She and 150 of her friends made Joy Care Bears and delivered them to area hospitals. They've given more than 3,600 bears to cancer patients to ease their minds and boost their spirits as they go through their treatment. A community has been formed because Joyce realized how powerful it was to have a broad base of support as she carved her path to health.

And finally, there's **Leanne Woodland**'s story. Her young son, Drew, was diagnosed with neuroblastoma. Surgery, chemo, and radiation proved no match for Drew's cancer. The cancer, however, proved no match for Leanne's determination to find a way to heal her son. Doctors told Leanne there was nothing more they could do for Drew. They then asked if she would subject her young son to clinical trials. Leanne chose to stop conventional treatment and heal her son with nutrition—and that was close to twenty years ago. Leanne is now a strong advocate for alternative health care, having firsthand experience with its success in saving her son's life.

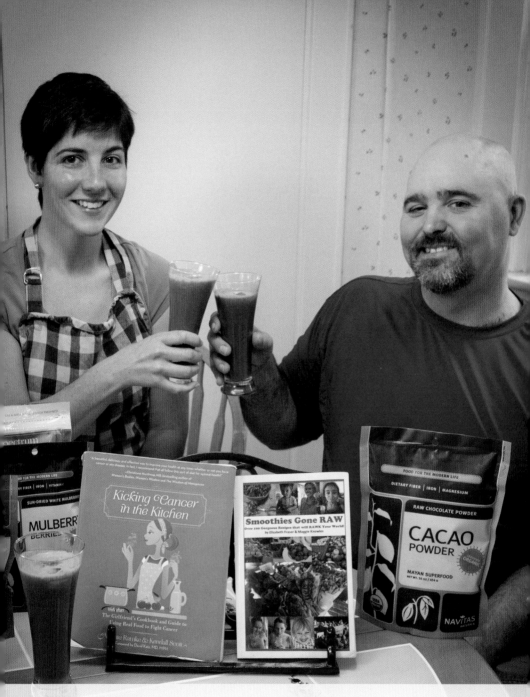

"I juice or blend smoothies almost every morning for breakfast, and continue to eat the colors of the rainbow throughout the day. I also continue on a monthly maintenance dose of vitamin C injection."

Diagnosis: Astrocytoma, brain cancer, stage II at first, then a year later stage III

Treatment: Brain surgery removed 90% of the tumor; within a year it grew back and the physician at the time felt it was a stage III, or possibly even a IV, but couldn't tell without surgery and taking a sample. Stuart couldn't complete the first cycle of chemo because it made him so sick. After six weeks of radiation, there was no success in tumor reduction.

What was the most important question you asked following your cancer diagnosis?

How did I get this?

How did you change your diet and/or lifestyle following your cancer diagnosis? At whose suggestion?

An alternative cancer physician suggested I change my lifestyle or the treatments were not going to work. Willpower and my wife helped me adjust to my new way of life with food. I went from not caring what I ate to caring about what I put in my body.

The hardest part of the change in diet was giving up all sugars, breads, and animal products. At that point, I took responsibility for my health. I switched to eating organic foods, and incorporated juicing raw vegetables and making green smoothies to increase the

Pictured: Stuart Cobb and his wife, Kristen Cobb

vegetables and fruit my doctor had recommended. Nuts and seeds became my new form of protein.

What treatment/lifestyle modification do you feel worked best for you? And why?

Definitely the less toxic treatment. Chemo was horrible, I just wanted to die while I was on it. It made me feel so sick. I turned to intravenous vitamin C and a strict diet regimen which consisted of increasing organic vegetables, fruits, and alkalizing rich foods, while decreasing consumption of animal products. Vitamins and an alkalizing water system were also recommended. Healing with natural foods and vitamin C had no side effects—that is, unless feeling good is a side effect. It was a win-win!

What do you wish you had known when you were diagnosed? What advice do you have for someone receiving a cancer diagnosis today?

That there are other ways to cure cancer without having to be cut, poisoned or burned.

Environmental factors contribute to cancer.

Be your own advocate.

What did you learn from having cancer?

Cell phones can be dangerous devices. When something is not working in your body, it's time for Plan B. Sugar feeds cancer, and cancer cannot survive in an alkalizing body. Cancer is big business. People shouldn't take the easy way out with a pill; foods are healing. Traditional doctors are not always right, because food does matter. Cancer is curable!

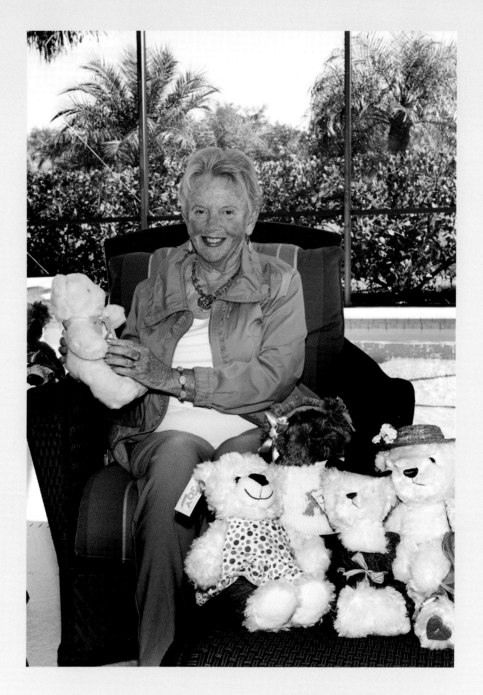

"If you allow it, cancer can take over your life in a negative way. I chose to learn from my battle and to turn it into a positive experience."

Diagnosis: Ovarian cancer

Treatment: When she was diagnosed at sixty-four, Joyce's treatment included surgery and chemotherapy followed by a plant-based diet and herbal supplements after recurrence.

What was the most important question you asked following your cancer diagnosis?

My husband and I were both overwhelmed by my initial diagnosis. Everything happened so fast: I was in surgery two weeks after the original diagnosis. I mainly remember asking how long the chemo treatments would last and whether there were any other options.

How did you change your diet and/or lifestyle following your cancer diagnosis?

I was initially diagnosed in February 2008 and went through six months of chemo following surgery. I had a recurrence in October 2009 and went through another six months of chemo.

When I had a recurrence in 2010, I decided not to have any more chemo. I started working with a nutritionist who specialized in cancer patients and began a plant-based diet.

What treatment do you continue to follow?

I visit my oncologist every six months, but have not needed any further tests or treatments from him. I continue to be on a plant-based diet with herbal supplements.

What treatment/lifestyle modification do you feel worked best for you? And why?

I have been cancer-free since I changed to a plant-based diet and added herbal supplements to boost my immune system. The biggest change that seems to have worked best for me has been eliminating dairy completely from my diet.

What did you learn from having cancer?

You need to try and take charge of your treatment plan as much as possible. Most oncologists seem to have tunnel vision in fighting ovarian cancer and in thinking that chemo treatments are the only way to fight it. There are other options to try!

I also learned that you can't battle cancer alone—you need a strong support team and the power of prayer to get you through the tough times.

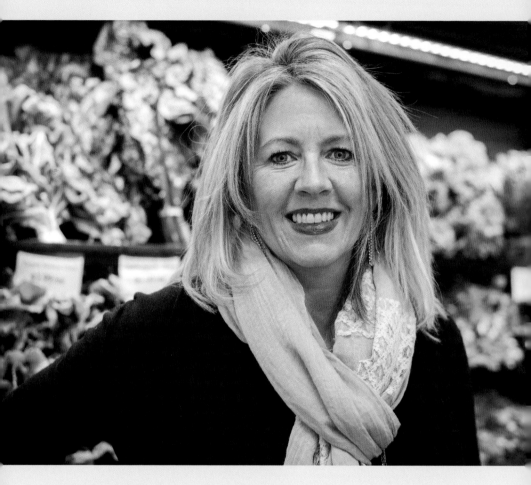

"People need to take full ownership of their illness, and if they are too sick to think clearly, they need an advocate to come alongside them until they are strong enough to embrace their natural cure."

On December 10th, 1992, Leanne Woodland's son Drew was diagnosed with stage IV cancer: neuroblastoma. He was only eighteen months old. His cancer was spread throughout his entire body. A grapefruit-sized tumor with finger-like tentacles attached to his kidneys, liver, pancreas and spine as well as throughout his mesenteric artery. Drew's aorta was also encased within the tumor mass.

Treatment: After one and a half years of intense "adult dosage" chemo and radiation, and multiple unsuccessful surgeries to remove the mass, Drew was sent home to die.

What was the most important question you asked following your son's cancer diagnosis?

I asked the team of doctors what our options were in curing Drew's cancer. They informed me that neuroblastoma is the deadliest form of childhood cancer. They followed that by explaining we had two options: "Do nothing and your son will die within four to six months or do chemo and radiation treatments and he'll have a 50% chance of survival."

How did you change Drew's diet and/or lifestyle following his cancer diagnosis? At whose suggestion?

I came across a book that spoke of building up the body's immune system to heal disease. I learned that by using whole, organic foods, organic juices and natural supplements, we could turbo-boost

Drew's immune system to fight the cancer. I immediately had our oncologist place a G-tube in Drew's abdomen so we could bolus-feed the organic juices and ground-up supplements into his body, bypassing the "battle" of trying to get a now almost three-year-old boy to eat the volume of foods and organic juices to build up his immune system.

What treatment/lifestyle modification do you feel worked best for your son? And why?

Drew was healed within six months of starting his alternative cancer treatment! Yes, he was cancer-free. His doctors were astounded! His healthy cells had attacked the tumor, destroying the finger-like cancerous tentacles and forcing the tumor mass to encase itself in a protein barrier, forever imprisoned and dying. Because of his miraculous healing, Drew's oncologist implemented, to the best of her ability, alternative cancer treatments.

What treatment(s) does Drew continue to follow?

An organic whole foods diet when affordable, supplements, cannabis oil (50/50 blend of CBD and THC), and baking soda.

What do you wish you had known when your son was diagnosed? What advice do you have for someone receiving a cancer diagnosis today?

I wrote two books detailing the pain, the program we used, and shared our passions to alert others of their options. What I failed to realize at that time and while writing my two books was this: When I read the initial book on healing, immediately my heart and mind had total belief that it would heal him because it all made so much sense to my spirit/higher self. The hope, faith, belief and, most importantly, the energy in our household changed from one of preparing for death to one of love, life, laughter and inspiration.

Today, after evolving and maturing into a deeper understanding of the power of our thoughts and the power of our feelings, I am even more convinced that what healed Drew was pure intention, positive thought, and a belief in what we were doing, coupled with using whole organic foods and natural supplements to build his immune system.

What did you learn from helping your son heal his cancer?

The most important thing I've learned in the past twenty-plus years while researching and working to educate people on their options is that there are hundreds—no, millions—of people desperately seeking a cure and they need an advocate. They need help, hope, healing, insights, information, resources in their community, and simple truths about how nature was designed, along with the human body, to cure disease *if* we give ourselves, our bodies the proper tools. Sadly, I also learned very quickly that there is a system of control out there to keep people from knowing about real cures for many diseases, including cancer, and that if anyone tries to break that system, The System will try to break them.

What else would you like to share?

The United States is not a friendly country when it comes to natural cures. The medical profession in this country is "birthed" to sell pharmaceutical drugs, and science continues to segment parts of the body as if one organ does not impact another. Natural cures treat the whole person, the whole illness, and the whole body.

People need to also understand that their emotional well-being has a very powerful impact on their body and its ability to develop disease or fight it. Holding on to negative energy, being around negative people or environments, and allowing stress to continually overtake them will cause the body's immune system to break down. Rid your life of negativity, including your own self-talk. The emerging science of psychoneuroimmunology has proven that our bodies become literally addicted to negativity and stress on a cellular level. I like to ask people if they personally know someone who seems angry or negative all the time, even when something good happens in their life . . . somehow they turn it into a negative. Often I see heads nod or hear a resounding "Yes!" I'll then explain that the person they are thinking of has—on a cellular/biological level—literally become addicted to the chemicals those harmful emotions produce in the body. People understand that science immediately. The truth always resonates with the spirit.

In 2013, Drew graduated from college with honors as a Film and Photography major at Montana State University in Bozeman. He won the Bruce Moore Award, which recognizes students who not only complete their degree successfully but also help others along the way to complete their degree projects. The award recipient is chosen by peers and college professors. He's a creative and quirky genius. He is an astounding artist, a keen photographer, and a budding filmmaker. Anyone who has had the pleasure of knowing Drew knows their life has been impacted in a very special and positive way.

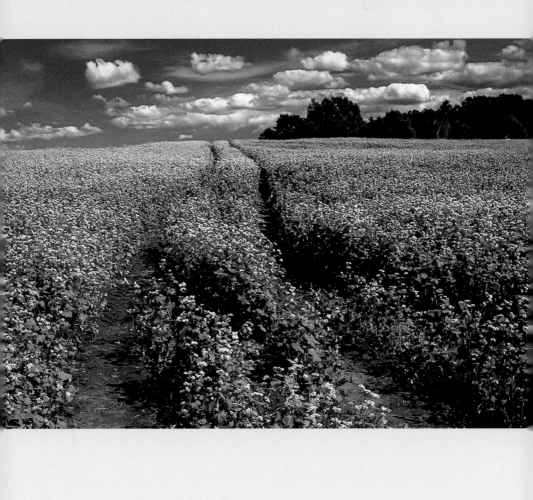

— 3 —

Plants to the Rescue

T HE WOMEN IN this chapter refused to let their cancer diagnoses take control of their lives. Instead, they chose to combat their cancer, in part, by changing up their diets and adding more plants to their plates.

The women in **Brenda Cobb**'s family had a long-standing relationship with cancer. Rather than following in the footsteps of family members who lost their lives to cancer, Brenda made the bold decision to decline the recommended surgery, chemo, and radiation. She combined an organic, vegan, raw, living-food diet with a variety of complementary therapies and has remained cancer-free for more than fifteen years. Excited to share her experience with others, Brenda founded the Living Foods Institute, where she and her staff teach healthy lifestyle programs. She has also written several books that describe her journey and inspire those who want to explore a living-foods lifestyle.

Kathryn Lorusso took advantage of the skills she developed as a journalist to research the treatment options that were available to her. She credits changing her diet with allowing her to recover quickly from both surgery and radiation treatments. Anxious to spread the knowledge she gained during her cancer treatment about the power of nutrition, Kathryn became a Food for Life Instructor through the Physicians Committee for Responsible Medicine program. She teaches classes on diabetes, weight loss, cancer prevention, and a kids' cooking class—always encouraging her students to follow her example and take charge of their health.

Elizabeth Petty was following a treatment plan mapped out by her health care team when she learned about the benefits of eating a raw foods diet. Elizabeth explored incorporating raw food into her diet by spending time at Hippocrates Health Institute. She was so enthralled with the raw foods lifestyle, in fact, that after healing her cancer she opened a restaurant, Elizabeth's Gone Raw (Washington, DC). The restaurant serves gourmet raw food and has allowed Elizabeth to expose a new audience to delicious and healthy raw food. Elizabeth's Gone Raw has been greeted with great success and has expanded its hours and offerings in response to customer demand.

Diagnosed with cancer at age twenty-seven, **Kendall Scott** took some time to envision how she'd like her future to look following her cancer treatment. She enrolled in a health coaching program offered by the Institute for Integrative Nutrition and changed her diet and lifestyle. As she says on her website, she and her business partner "adopted a 'food as medicine' philosophy." This mindset helped Kendall identify her mission to "empower, inspire and educate women—whether facing cancer or not—in finding their food groove and making positive lifestyle choices so they can feel stronger, healthier and happier."

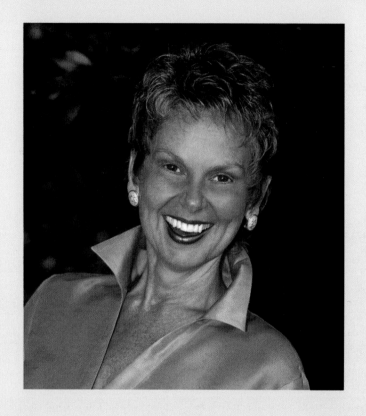

"Fear blocks healing. Faith speeds up healing.
Believe in the power of healing and give thanks."

Diagnosis: Breast and cervical cancer

Treatment: Brenda's family had a long history of breast, cervical, and uterine cancer. When she was diagnosed at age fifty in 1999, Brenda rejected her doctor's advice—no surgery, chemo, or radiation for her.

What was the most important question you asked following your cancer diagnosis?

I prayed and asked God to direct me in the right way to naturally heal my body.

How did you change your diet and/or lifestyle following your cancer diagnosis?

I stopped eating animal products, dairy, sugar, and processed food, and began eating organic raw and living (sprouted) foods. I did colonics, enemas, and wheatgrass implants. I also focused on emotional healing, forgiveness, and stress management.

What treatment/lifestyle modification do you feel worked best for you?

I continue to eat organic raw and living foods and include massages, reflexology, acupuncture, and chiropractic adjustments in my health management routine.

What do you wish you had known when you were diagnosed? What advice do you have for someone receiving a cancer diagnosis today?

I wish I had realized how much food matters to a healthy body and that eating lots of animal protein is damaging to the body.

I advise people not to feel pressured by doctors to rush into doing surgery and treatments they don't feel good about. I encourage them to investigate alternative, natural ways to heal.

What did you learn from having cancer?

I learned that I created cancer by holding on to negative emotions and not paying attention to my diet. My stressful lifestyle resulted in an environment where cancer could easily grow in my body.

What else would you like to share?

The body was created to heal itself and it can do that beautifully when it is given the nutrition and support it needs. It is never too late, no matter how far advanced the disease, as long as you're willing to make the necessary lifestyle changes.

Brenda Cobb founded the Living Foods Institute in 1999 (www.livingfoodsinstitute.com, 800-844-9876).

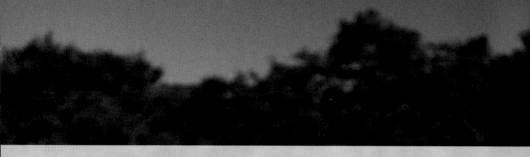

"My advice to someone would be to take your health into your own hands. Do not walk into a doctor's office and hear the diagnosis and treatment plan without realizing you need to take an active part."

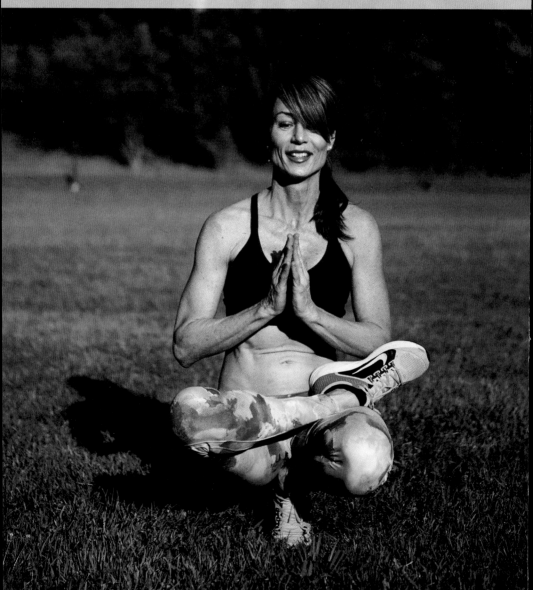

Kathryn Lorusso

Diagnosis: Stage I breast cancer
Treatment: A plant-based diet, lumpectomy, and twenty-five rounds of radiation

What was the most important question you asked following your cancer diagnosis?

I asked, "Am I going to survive?" My doctor immediately said yes and then I asked, "What happens next?"

What treatment/lifestyle modification do you feel worked best for you?

I took a collaborative approach and worked with my "healing team" of surgeon, radiologist, and oncologist. I asked six million questions, offered my research to them, and we all settled on a healing plan that I could live with and that made sense to me. I even collaborated on the angle and depth of the radiation beam, the anesthesia for the surgery, and the follow-up drugs with my oncologist (I decided to take *none*). There was nothing I wasn't a part of, and I loved that.

What did you learn from having cancer?

I still consider cancer one of the best things that ever happened to me. It opened my eyes to the miraculous power of a plate of veggies, fruits, grains and beans. I began cooking for myself and others and realized my refrigerator was my new medicine cabinet.

I could play the biggest role in my own healing and health every day!

I am my own best health advocate, and I love teaching others how to claim their power and work with their doctors. I was moving through my life at a faster and faster speed and ignoring important signals from my body. Cancer slowed me down so that I now see and feel all of those signals.

I work with my body now and believe that everything I put in my mouth is either healing or hurting me. I choose my food accordingly! I'm also looking forward to teaching the Physicians Committee for Responsible Medicine cancer series cooking classes to my oncologist's patients in the future.

What treatment(s) do you continue to follow?

I am not following a "treatment plan" with my doctors but I do have six-month checkups and blood work with my oncologist. She is a wonderful, kind, caring human being who takes an inordinate amount of time with me and is very interested in my diet. She has finally agreed that I am not a candidate for Tamoxifen or other invasive procedures (ovary removal) and that my diet is nothing short of miraculous. The last time I saw her, she said, "You are going to live a very long time!"

What advice do you have for someone receiving a cancer diagnosis today?

I am a former journalist, so researching is my nature. I immediately found my macrobiotic counselor and changed my diet. This helped me recover very quickly from surgery, with barely a scar. The radiation treatments were never a problem, either.

In fact, I never felt better! I sailed into the hospital every morning before work, slid into the machine, got zapped and then did a full day of work at school. I never felt tired, never had scarring, never turned red or peeled . . . never had a second of side effects whatsoever. I was eating miso and seaweed and tons of veggies and grains and was ecstatic to be alive and moving through my cancer diagnosis.

Tell the doctor(s) what would make you comfortable or uncomfortable. What do you need? What do you not understand? If your diagnosing doctor doesn't take the time to work with you, *find another doctor*. You deserve good care and you need to be comfortable in order to stay positive and heal.

Doctors are also not trained in medical school to understand the healing powers of vegetables, fruits, grains, and beans. They are highly trained to treat symptoms. Thank God for them! But you cannot expect them to tell you how to eat or even that eating differently will help you. There are nutrition experts to help with that part. Find one and get going!

What else would you like to share?

Even though the word "cancer" is one of the scariest words you may ever hear, facing your own mortality does not have to be a horrible event. It can be liberating! We are all going to die, but isn't it great to know that you have very real options to prolong your life and feel fantastic in the meantime? The vegan lifestyle is becoming more and more mainstream and easier and easier to adopt. The success stories are everywhere!

Kathryn can be found online at www.thankfulfoods.com.

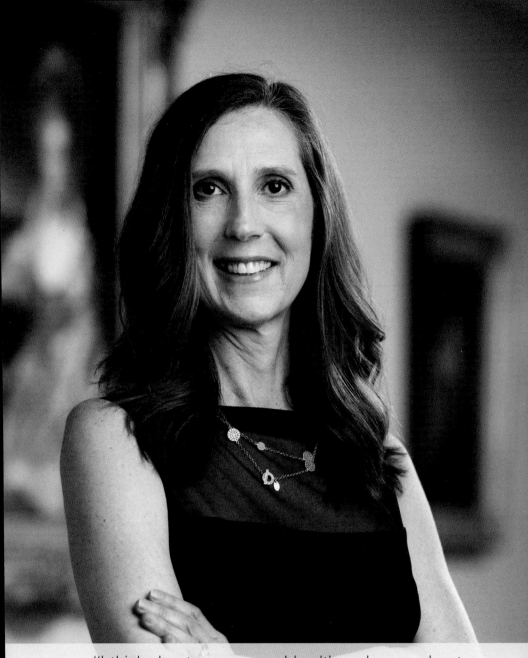

"I think about my personal health and more about how I can make a difference in the world. What can I do in small ways to change the way that people choose to eat? I'm even more blessed than I realized. Being in the food industry gives me a platform to share something that's become a passion for me."

Diagnosis: Stage IIa breast cancer
Treatment: Surgery, radiation, chemotherapy, raw foods diet,
a variety of complementary care at Hippocrates Health Institute
including sauna and yoga

What was the most important question you asked following your cancer diagnosis?

I don't know that any one question stands out for me. Critical to my treatment was reading and researching treatment options.

How did you change your diet and/or lifestyle following your cancer diagnosis?

While I was undergoing conventional treatment, I read *Crazy Sexy Cancer Tips* by Kris Carr. This opened my eyes to treatment options, and I contacted Dr. Brian Clement of Hippocrates Health Institute.

After talking with Brian, I went to Hippocrates Health Institute for three weeks. This was a life-changing experience for me. I adopted a vegan, raw foods diet which includes eighty ounces of green juices; I eliminated fruit from my diet for three years. While recuperating and healing at Hippocrates, I came up with the idea of opening a raw foods restaurant.

What treatment/lifestyle modification do you feel worked best for you? And why?

The vegan, raw foods diet allowed me to endure rigorous medical treatment—five surgeries, chemotherapy, and radiation—and was key in restoring my health.

What treatment(s) do you continue to follow?

I continue to follow a vegan diet, 80% to 90% of which is raw.

What do you wish you had known when you were diagnosed?

I wish I had known that there are many paths to health. I feel like I acted impulsively in choosing a treatment plan. In hindsight, I realize I could have taken more time to make that decision.

What advice do you have for someone receiving a cancer diagnosis today?

Look at this health challenge as an opportunity to change your life for the better.

Slow down and breathe. Read, talk to people who have had cancer, and educate yourself before making choices.

Take an active role in determining your treatment plan. You are part of your medical team. My oncologist was skeptical when I incorporated raw foods into my treatment; at the end of the treatment, however, she was impressed with how well I responded to the treatment, which we attribute at least partly to my raw diet.

What did you learn from having cancer?

Having cancer provided me with the opportunity to experience a whole new lifestyle. Opening a raw foods restaurant (Elizabeth's Gone Raw - elizabethsgoneraw.com) has fulfilled me in a way I never dreamed possible.

What else would you like to share?

I feel as though initially I changed my lifestyle because of my health challenge; now because I've lived this lifestyle for so long, I feel like there's a much richer spiritual and emotional aspect to it. I now have a broader concern for humanity and ethical treatment of animals. What impact does diet have on our culture and what role do I play in that? How can I educate people without judging choices that people make? Change happens through education.

I've been able to develop spiritually and recognize the importance of change culturally. Even small change has an enormous impact on the environment, on the way that people feel, on people's behavior, by elevating consciousness and being more thoughtful about food and lifestyle choices. There are lessons to be learned from ancient cultures when you realize how much thoughtfulness goes into agriculture. What does it mean to eat with a friend, with your family? We need to put our hands in the dirt, get them dirty, and have a conversation over a good meal.

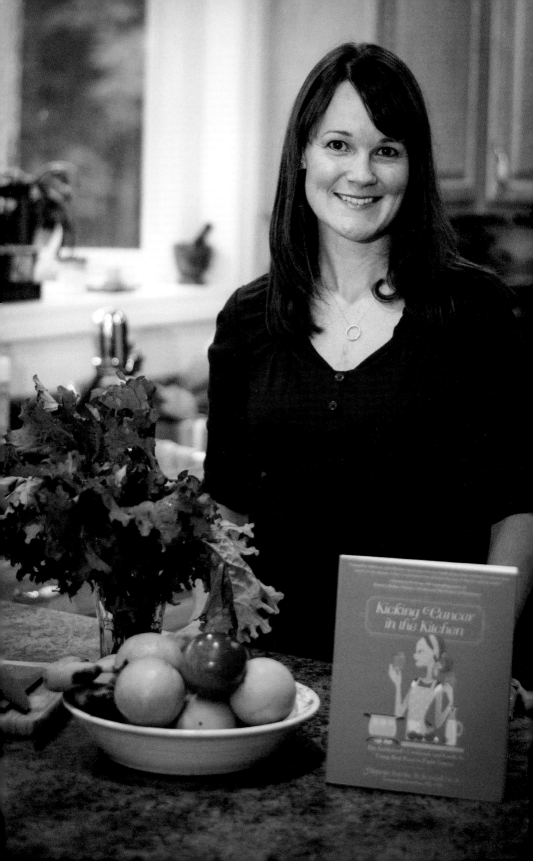

Kendall Scott, CHHC

Diagnosis: Stage IIa Hodgkin's lymphoma
Treatment: When she was diagnosed at age twenty-seven in 2008, Kendall's treatment included surgery and chemotherapy.

What was the most important question you asked following your cancer diagnosis?

What can I do to help fight the cancer and cope with treatment side effects? Specifically, should I eat better?

How did you change your diet and/or lifestyle following your cancer diagnosis?

I focused on adding in whole foods, more plant foods, crowding out the processed and refined food and sugar, and on reducing animal food. The first step was to add more leafy greens. To this day, I feel eating these veggies makes the biggest difference in my overall health.

My aunt had recently become a board-certified health coach and offered guidance in how to make changes in my diet. I then continued researching on my own and ended up attending the Institute for Integrative Nutrition to learn more.

"Getting a cancer diagnosis doesn't have to be the end. In fact, for me, it was a whole new beginning to a completely different and far better way of life."

What treatment/lifestyle modification do you feel worked best for you? And why?

Eating and living more naturally—that means eating whole, plant-based foods as well as reducing chemicals in the home and personal hygiene. Perhaps even more importantly, becoming more connected to my body, how I'm feeling on all levels, and learning how to make improvements naturally whenever possible to support overall health and wellness.

What do you wish you had known when you were diagnosed? What advice do you have for someone receiving a cancer diagnosis today?

I wish I had known that what we do, how we live, what we eat—it all makes a huge difference when it comes to our health. We have more power than we often believe in living a long, healthy, happy life.

I would also advise people to look at many different options for treatment—from conventional, to completely natural and everything in between. Get second opinions, see a naturopathic doctor or integrative physician, in addition to an oncologist. While it may feel overwhelming, you will likely be much happier with the outcome.

What did you learn from having cancer?

I learned so much about listening to my body and eating well through my cancer experience, but I also learned what is truly important in my life—the people I love, good health.

Just enjoying the little things, which, in the end, really are the "big" things: holding my children, snuggling with my husband, walking barefoot in the grass, laughing until my stomach hurts, spending time with family and friends, digging in my garden, helping someone in need, running on the beach . . . those are the things that bring me joy and make life so very worth living.

Kendall Scott, CHHC, is a health coach, author of *Kicking Cancer in the Kitchen*, and can be found online at The Kicking Kitchen (thekickingkitchen.com).

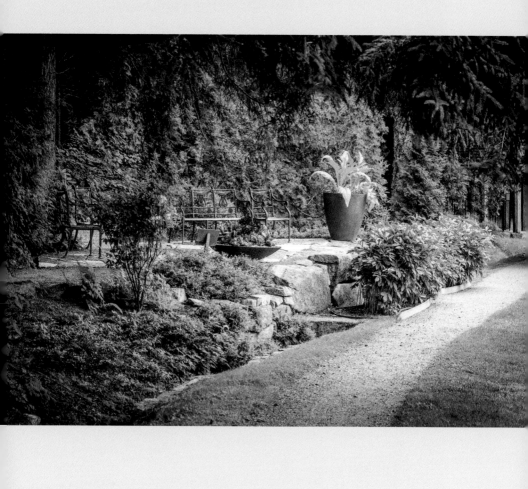

4

When East Meets West

MACROBIOTICS (MEANING "LARGE or great life") was introduced to the United States in California by George Ohsawa, the father of macrobiotics. Two of his students, Michio and Aveline Kushi, spread their knowledge of macrobiotics to the East Coast through the Kushi Institute.

In his book *Macrobiotics for Dummies*, Verne Varona defines macrobiotics as "large or great life" and describes the practice of macrobiotics as "a philosophy for dynamic living. It provides practical and inspirational tools for enhancing and balancing health, elevating judgment, stabilizing moods, improving mental clarity, increasing intuitive sensitivity and fortifying your internal flow of energy."

Each of the people you'll meet in this chapter incorporated the macrobiotic lifestyle into their treatment.

Judith Dean MacKenney underwent one chemotherapy treatment before discovering that her doctors expected her to die from some form of chemo. She learned about macrobiotics and, along with her husband, Larry, embraced this lifestyle. Now more than twenty years later, Judy is a healthy, well-respected macrobiotic counselor and teacher.

Gina Paterno Villalobos also turned to macrobiotics to heal her cancer. Like Judy, Gina had the full support of her husband as she navigated her path to health. Gina took the best the East and West had to offer, incorporating Western medicine in her treatment. She made a conscious decision, with the help of her husband, to look at life through a positive lens during her treatment. She was aware that she had a choice of whether to be positive or negative; being positive spurred her forward toward health.

John Watson had his sister by his side every step of the way on his journey to health. Marlene Watson-Tara is a macrobiotic counselor and helped John take control of his life and health by taking control of his diet. He decided to stop abusing his body and adopted a macrobiotic lifestyle to ease the stress his diet had placed on his body. John's relationship with his sister took on a new meaning as he healed his cancer.

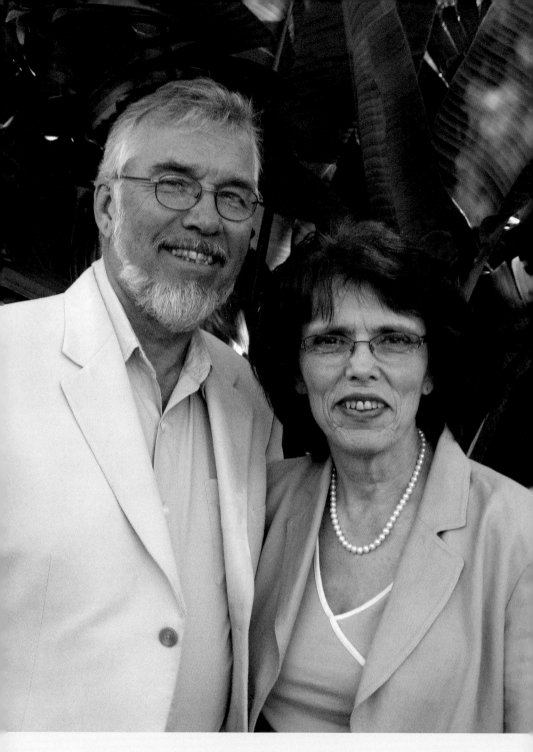

"Embrace your faith, family, and friends for support."

Judith Dean MacKenney

Diagnosis: Stage II to stage IV non-Hodgkin's lymphoma
Treatment: One-drug protocol of Chlorambucil chemotherapy,
then adopted a macrobiotic lifestyle.

What was the most important question you asked following your cancer diagnosis?

Doctors expressed that my condition was inoperable and incurable. They recommended a one-drug protocol of Chlorambucil, a non-curative, oral chemotherapy. My question to them was, "What would I die of?" They told me I'd die of a stronger chemotherapy, eventually breaking down my immune system. This was a stage IV terminal illness to them.

How did you change your diet and/or lifestyle following your cancer diagnosis? At whose suggestion?

A healer inspired me to seek out Dr. Bernie Siegel, who founded a support group for exceptional cancer patients in New Haven, Connecticut. Meeting with this group of people with similar conditions in a safe, positive setting was paramount to my healing.

Bernie offered a lending library on alternative and complementary therapies. There I discovered *The Cancer Prevention Diet* by Michio Kushi, which changed my life. During my illness, I searched for answers to my health problems and Michio Kushi's

Pictured: Judith Dean MacKenney and her husband, Larry MacKenney words of encouragement were the first offer of a solution. I met with Dr. Marc van Cauwenberghe, a prominent macrobiotic counselor who came highly recommended. He suggested I change my diet and lifestyle using macrobiotics and that, by doing so, I could heal myself.

What treatment/lifestyle modification do you feel worked best for you? And why?

The macrobiotic diet and lifestyle, utilizing natural home remedies, whole foods, organic grains, beans, vegetables, and sea vegetables cleansed and healed my body. I stopped ingesting meat, dairy, sugar, sugar products, and sugar substitutes and began detoxifying. My blood work improved immensely after three to four months. My anemia disappeared, and I experienced energy that I hadn't felt in years, along with a return to peaceful sleep.

I also took daily walks with my friends (deep-breathing oxygen and blowing out toxins), chewed my food thoroughly to allow the enzymes to help in the digestive process, listened to joyful music, and laughed at comedy video tapes with friends and family.

What treatment(s) do you continue to follow?

I continue to follow the organic macrobiotic whole and plant food philosophies. This has eliminated the need for any and all other treatments.

What do you wish you had known when you were diagnosed? What advice do you have for someone receiving a cancer diagnosis today?

I wish I had known that I could have healed without using chemotherapy. What we ingest creates great impact on our healing and wellness. In a time of crisis, we get caught up in fear and panic.

You must be willing to change, to get educated, to seek professionals who can support natural ways of healing, to get inspired, to seek group support, and to take the time to cleanse and rebuild your body, mind, and spirit.

What did you learn from having cancer?

I learned that cancer does not have to be a death sentence. It's a wake-up call. It's important to make the time and effort to learn well, cook well, and assume responsibility for your own health, instead of leaving it in the hands of others. Being grateful for living each day to the fullest, for family and friends, for being at peace in nature. I've learned that quality of life is the important issue, not quantity of years.

What else would you like to share?

You must believe that you have the power and the courage to heal. Hope is the most important emotion. It creates possibilities to succeed. Macrobiotics meant hope and freedom from illness to me. We did a daring thing during my illness. We moved to a warmer climate, which allowed my body to relax and heal. My dear family and friends were paramount in my healing process with their encouragement, love, and kindnesses.

My husband Larry, my soul mate, stood by me unconditionally. He intuitively suggested, then navigated "our healing journey to Florida." It is our joy and privilege to continue to inspire and serve groups and individuals seeking wellness and optimal health!

Judy offers counseling and teaching through Harmony Haven Healing Arts (www.harmonyhavenhealingarts.com, judymackenney@gmail.com).

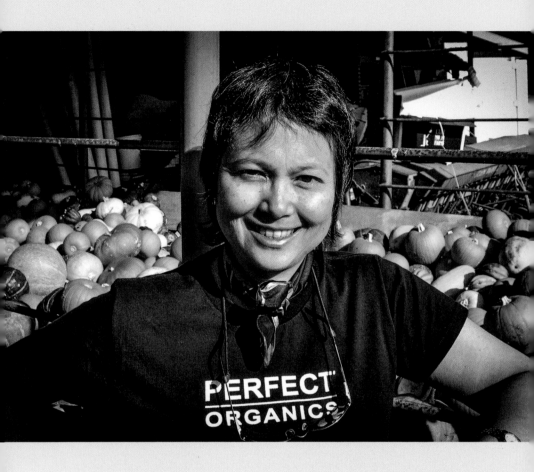

"It's incredibly important to be conscious of how you look at things—and how you choose to look at things. Your outlook, attitude, and approach to life affects your mind and your body, and can help you to overcome everything."

GINA PATERNO VILLALOBOS

Diagnosis: Stage IIIc breast cancer
Treatment: Gina's health plan combined the best that Eastern and Western philosophies have to offer. In addition to adopting a macrobiotic approach to diet and lifestyle, she had a lumpectomy, radiation, and chemical ovarian suppression for five to six years due to her high-risk profile.

What was the most important question you asked following your cancer diagnosis?

I would say it wasn't any one question that was most important, but continuing to ask questions about every aspect of my treatment. I'm actually surprised that I intuitively knew exactly what I needed to do.

I focused on what needed to get done and what I had to do. I immediately started researching and took charge. I put all my effort and energy into understanding my diagnosis and my treatment options and became an advocate for myself. By noon of the day following my diagnosis, I had lined up appointments with four of the best breast surgeons in the country and three oncologists—somehow I got on their calendars.

For me it was all about focusing in and putting my whole being into what needed to be done next. I completely owned my treatment and researched every element of my treatment so that I could understand everything I was going through. All of the changes I was making were making a positive impact on my mind, body, and spirit.

How did you change your diet and/or lifestyle following your cancer diagnosis?

I knew it was time to make a change in my life. I had ignored signals from my body for too long. Intuitively, I felt my diet and lifestyle had contributed to my illness. It was time to take charge of my health and look after Number One: Me!

The moment I found out I had thirteen nodes positive (after a second surgery), my risk profile changed completely. I was depressed for two hours, and then my entire outlook on life changed. I surrounded myself with positivity and love. I wore happy colors, watched happy movies, spent time with people who were supportive of me. Every night I wrote a journal entry about three things I was grateful for in my life. My husband joined me in this choice to be positive and said: "We are going to love this cancer away." And that is what we've done by taking everything one step at a time.

I immersed myself in studying the holistic, macrobiotic approach to diet and lifestyle, which incorporates traditional wisdom and longevity practices of traditional cultures around the world and the Eastern philosophy of energy balance within ourselves and our environment.

To make sure I was learning as much as I could about the connection between diet and lifestyle and what causes disease, I trained at the Kushi Institute Center for Natural Healing and earned certification as a macrobiotic instructor. I also earned certification in food therapy from the Natural Gourmet Institute for Food & Health and in plant-based nutrition from Cornell University.

Incorporating holistic modalities, including a meditation-based stress reduction course, acupuncture, reiki, yoga, and Qigong, was also part of my treatment plan.

What treatment/lifestyle modification do you feel worked best for you? And why?

To this day, I feel that my total change in diet was one of the most important things. With that, of course, came spiritual development.

By following a balanced macrobiotic diet and way of living while being more holistic, I feel the healthiest that I have ever been! I'm also cancer-free and no longer need my hypertension medication (which I was prescribed prior to the breast cancer, another one of those body signals that I chose to ignore!). I've dramatically lowered my cholesterol and have managed to lose 50 pounds in the process, and to maintain my weight loss, a first ever!

Reducing the stress in my life was also important. When my company restructured, I took the opportunity to change my career and follow a less stressful career path. Who I was and what I did became one.

What treatment(s) do you continue to follow?

I continue to look at things positively. It's how I choose to be and to live. Doing the things that matter to me most and keeping a positive attitude overall are key to my lifestyle.

I also continue to follow a macrobiotic diet and lifestyle while including meditation, yoga, and Qigong in my daily life.

What advice do you have for someone receiving a cancer diagnosis today?

1. It's all in the head—your attitude—*how you choose to look at things.*

2. Don't get too far ahead of yourself: take your cancer journey day by day. You'll have some good days. You'll

have some bad days. The key is to make sure you're moving in the right direction.

3. Surround yourself with positivity and let go of any energy drains.

What did you learn from having cancer?

I'm grateful that I took the time to be my own health advocate. While my husband supported me fully during this journey, it was important for me to do the research about the treatment options that were available to me.

I'm grateful for living; I'm being grateful for life, for what the universe has to offer, for the small things, flowers, sunrise, sunset. Find something to be grateful for every day and appreciate life.

I just took charge, choosing to be positive to move forward.

I was given a big gift—the gift of a high-risk breast cancer diagnosis. As soon as I learned my diagnosis, I accepted it. I was never in denial or angry. I simply researched and moved forward every day. There was a fundamental shift in how I thought and acted from that day forward.

My life has changed so much since I was diagnosed with cancer. I had been working six or seven days a week and was exhausted. I took this opportunity to find a new way of life that fulfills me. My work life is in sync with my personal life, and that makes all the difference in the world to me.

What else would you like to share?

The importance of choosing a life of positivity is absolutely key. There's a lot of research on happiness and the important role it plays in our lives; a lot of the things I did, I did intuitively, and now they've become habits for me.

By helping myself, I was also able to help others.

Gina is now The Organic Coach® (www.theorganiccoach. com).

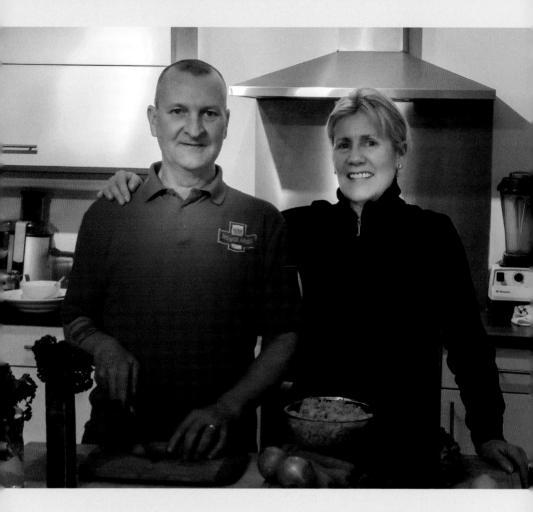

"The biggest form of mass destruction to human health lies at the end of your fork, and people need to take responsibility for their own health."

Diagnosis: Prostate cancer, metastasized to lymph nodes in stomach
Treatment: Estrogen injections

What was the most important question you asked following your cancer diagnosis?

Is it terminal?

How did you change your diet and/or lifestyle following your cancer diagnosis? At whose suggestion?

My sister, Marlene Watson-Tara, is a Macrobiotic Counsellor. She changed my diet 180 degrees—from a big meat, dairy, and sugar diet with lots of cakes and biscuits to a macrobiotic diet.

What treatment/lifestyle modification do you feel worked best for you? And why?

As Marlene explained, she was going to be removing the nutritional stress from my body by changing my diet to a whole foods, plant-based diet to allow for the amazing fact that we are a self-healing organism and the body would then start to come back into balance. She also explained that cancer is a disease of excess.

Pictured: John Watson and his sister, Marlene Watson-Tara

What treatment(s) do you continue to follow?

Estrogen injections, one every three months.

What do you wish you had known when you were diagnosed? What advice do you have for someone receiving a cancer diagnosis today?

The fact that only 3% of cancers are due to gene factors. Marlene tells me constantly that genes may load the gun, but lifestyle pulls the trigger.

What did you learn from having cancer?

That for most of my life I have abused my body with the typical Western diet.

What else would you like to share?

I wish my sister and her work would become famous so she can help educate the world about the fallacy that diet cannot control disease.

Marlene has a friend who works in the oncology department of a hospital in Portugal where she teaches, and she tells her that there is no way the results I had would come solely from these [estrogen] injections. My prostate-specific antigen (PSA) was 480. After seven weeks of Marlene cooking for me it, was 7.9, and it is now 2.6.

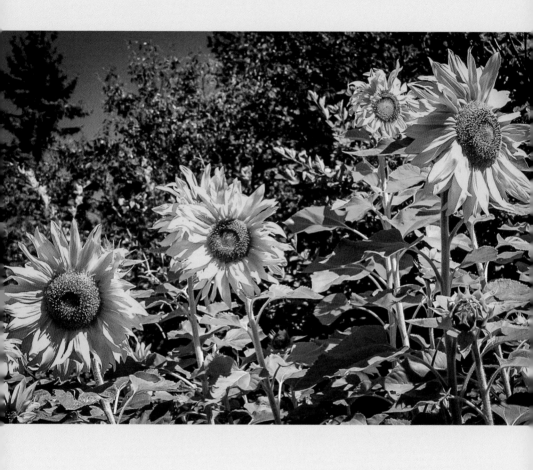

5

Conventional Treatment and Complementary/ Alternative Medicine

CANCER PATIENTS CAN include a variety of complementary and alternative therapies in their treatment plans. Sometimes the patients are on their own to include these elements in their treatment; sometimes the medical facility provides suggestions for inclusion in the treatment plan.

Dr. Dena Mendes became an advocate for her health and added a battery of complementary care elements to her treatment. In addition to working with doctors, Dena relied on her intuition. She added yoga, meditation, breathing exercises, Qigong, dance, and spiritual connection to her treatment plan. As her health improved, her reliance on her intuition grew. Dena also wrote a book documenting her experience with cancer and passing on her lessons learned. She encourages her patients to be strong advocates for themselves. Asking questions in a timely manner is important—having as much information as soon as possible is important when making decisions about your treatment.

Christina Parrish was diagnosed with pancreatic cancer and told that she had approximately six months to live. Knowing that she had a lot more living to do, Chris contacted Cancer Treatment Centers of America. After more tests and consults with a health care team at one of their facilities, Chris and her team put a plan together that involved conventional and complementary care. Chris has become a fierce advocate for pancreatic cancer patients. She founded a nonprofit organization, The Purple Iris, "to raise awareness, educate, support, and give hope to individuals and families affected by Pancreatic Cancer." She continues to share her life experiences on social media outlets, reaching out to others going through cancer treatment to lend a hand wherever she can.

Debbie Wylie also heard devastating information from her doctors: if she followed the recommended treatment plan, there was a 30% chance it would heal her cancer. The treatment was severe and could leave her eating through a feeding tube *if* she survived. Debbie conducted research and, with the support of friends, family, and community, opted to go to Mexico for treatment. Her treatment plan included a number of complementary elements that have left her healthy and energetic. She lives an active life filled with family and friends.

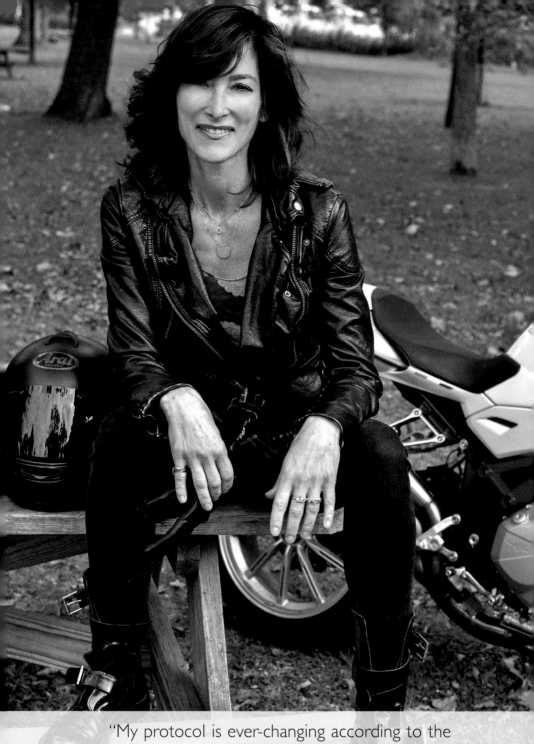

"My protocol is ever-changing according to the season and where I am at emotionally and physically."

Diagnosis: Stage I DCIS HER2/neu-positive

Treatment: The wrong chemotherapy (which Dena's doctors never told her was wrong, as it was their only "standard of care" at that time), Adriamycin 75 cytoxan chemo for estrogen-receptive tumors. Dena shared that the surgeon missed the pea-sized, totally encapsulated pre-cancerous tumor due to lack of a procedure called a frozen section that could have saved her from over a decade of metastasis.

What was the most important question you asked following your cancer diagnosis?

More important is what I didn't ask. I should have asked if they got clean margins immediately. Instead, I didn't know any better and the doctor didn't call me for five weeks to tell me I had "dirty margins."

Now that I know, I advise all my patients to make sure they request a frozen section. This procedure ensures that they get results immediately and that the doctor takes the extra time necessary to make sure he "gets all of the tumor." Whatever you do, do not wait around for the doctor to call you! Be pushy!

How did you change your diet and/or lifestyle following your cancer diagnosis?

I eliminated inflammation-causing foods like wheat and gluten, dairy, and sugar. I eat only grass-fed meats in small quantities. My diet includes greens, greens, and more greens! I eat according to my individual needs, not a one-size-fits-all plan. I am small, thin, and typically cold, so I could never live on raw food as that would be too damp and cold, creating a mold, fungal, yeast environment.

I added much more probiotics and alkalinizing protocols. Read my book *A Survivor's Guide to Kicking Cancer's Ass* to learn more about the foundation of all that ails us or heals us, our food! (See *www.denashealthyu.com.*)

I started to see a few natural doctors and mixed a bit of this one with a bit of that one. Throughout this process, I gained a new sense of myself and followed my very own intuitive prowess, which became keener as I cleared the inflammation out of my diet and off of my brain. I could see things more clearly. My intuition and intuitive prowess became spot-on!

What treatment/lifestyle modification do you feel worked best for you? And why?

I like to combine the emotional and physical components of dis-ease. I realized that I could eat greens until hell froze over, but if I didn't start working on my old stuck emotional anger, frustration, and resentment—all liver stuff—that I would continue to develop tumors on my right side, along the liver meridian channels. I took up Dahn yoga and started Qigong beating to clear old stuck emotional patterns. Using breathing, meditation, and a deeper spiritual connection to source helped me to heal.

What treatment(s) do you continue to follow?

Breathing, Dahn yoga, and tango dancing that helps me to get out of my ever-thinking mind, totally let go, and let someone else take the lead. I always use food as my first line of defense and a variety of unique supplements and protocols, depending on how I am feeling.

What do you wish you had known when you were diagnosed? What advice do you have for someone receiving a cancer diagnosis today?

I wish I had known to listen to the thermograph that showed no cancer because it was DCIS (ductal carcinoma in situ), which meant it was totally encapsulated and precancerous. Looking back, I wish I would have left it all alone and simply de-flamed myself with food, supplements, and emotional work. I had plenty of time: I didn't need to rush to do a thing, as the doctors wanted me to believe. I would *never* have taken the poisonous chemotherapy they gave me as "standard of care."

That is not to say that chemotherapy is never necessary for some people in the right setting, but mine was totally useless and not even the correct chemotherapy for the type of breast tumor I had been diagnosed with. So all it did was deplete my immune system when I needed it to fight for me. I'm so sad that the doctors never told me the truth or even gave me the option or choice.

What did you learn from having cancer?

I learned to heal others of any and all side effects from the ravages of chemotherapy, radiation and surgery hell! To let things go more, the dirty dishes, the angry words, the need to be right, and people who are not for my highest and best.

What else would you like to share?

Become an active participant in your health care process.

Gain an entirely new sense of your self.

Use your innate, God-given intuitive prowess.

Look for your gurus; they will come when you need them.

Be still, the answers will come in a dream, in a thought, or in another human being.

Do not simply follow like a lemming; you might follow right off a cliff.

Make no mistake about it; there is always an emotional component to every dis-ease!

There is no simpler equation than what you put in your mouth you get out! Food is your first line of defense! Food even changes your emotional well-being!

You will always have that *AHA* moment when all is said and done, even if it is the need to leave this earthly plane and move on to the next. There is nothing wrong with taking an adventure in passing over.

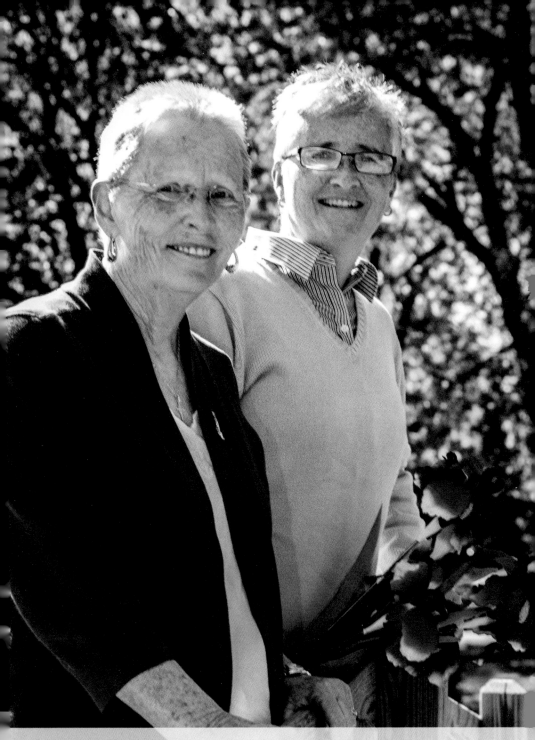

"Spread love and kindness. It matters."

CHRISTINA PARRISH

Diagnosis: Stage IV pancreatic cancer
Treatment: Intra-arterial therapy, FUDR administered with Leucovorin infusion for three and a half years

What was the most important question you asked following your cancer diagnosis?

What do I have to do to live (past the six months they gave me)? Where do I go that will give me a chance to fight and live?

How did you change your diet and/or lifestyle following your cancer diagnosis? At whose suggestion?

As soon as I found out, I stopped being in denial. I changed my diet to organic and anything that was good for me. With pancreatic cancer, it's difficult to digest food. I drank a lot of Ensure initially and juiced twice a day. Exercise continued to be a part of my routine.

What did you learn from having cancer?

I've learned so much! Mostly about myself—strength and determination. I learned that anything is possible.

Having cancer also taught me to enjoy the time I have with people. You never know how long they will be here. Everyone you meet has something to offer or teach you.

Pictured: Christina Parrish (r) and her mom, Phyllis Couch (l)

I don't carry my work home with me. I work for four hours a day, and then I go golfing, which has become my new passion. I even walk the golf course carrying my own bag. It's empowering for me to be able to do that. And when I'm not golfing, I'm at the beach. I'm like a kid: I'm not indoors until the sun comes down. I don't want to miss a thing. I work out and jog/walk about a half-mile, when I feel up to it. A couple of times, I've even played basketball. It's good for my body to do something different.

I've also started the Purple Iris Foundation, an initiative to raise awareness of pancreatic cancer (www.purpleirisfoundation.com and www.facebook.com/thepurpleirisfoundation). We've bought thousands of purple irises from the local garden club and planted them throughout the community. On Facebook, we have about 3,700 friends. It's my dream. I'd like to get it to take off and raise money for people who have pancreatic cancer and can't afford treatment.

What do you wish you had known when you were diagnosed? What advice do you have for someone receiving a cancer diagnosis today?

There is all kinds of information and resources available for those who have been diagnosed, but nothing prepares you for hearing the word "cancer." In my case, they said I had a mass on my pancreas and lesions on my liver. It was when I heard the word "oncologist"—that's when I started to cry.

I would advise anyone who gets a cancer diagnosis to get a second and third opinion.

What else would you like to share?

I really understood what "living" meant after I was told I had six months to live. It has been a gradual process, but learning to live in the moment is a spectacular thing.

Never take anyone or anything for granted.

Be thankful for everything, and never miss a chance to let the ones you love know how you feel!

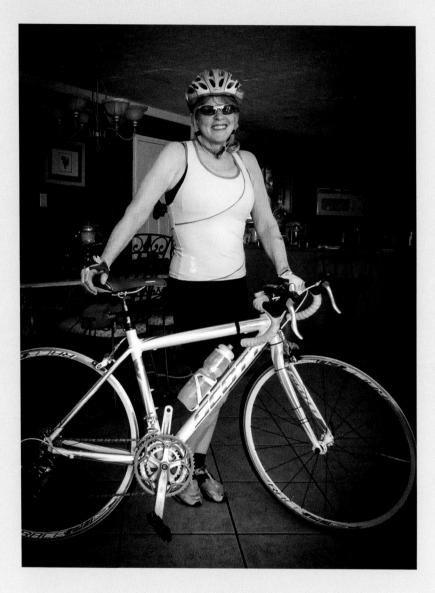

"Life is so worth living, and happiness is a choice!"

Diagnosis: Stage IV head/neck (tonsil) cancer
Treatment: Juicing, 70% raw diet, enzyme protocol, ozone treatments, coffee enemas, supplements, minimal chemotherapy and cobalt radiation, dental work

What was the most important question you asked following your cancer diagnosis?

What are my chances of survival? Experts told me I had a 30% chance to survive the crippling and severe treatment plan they offered: extensive chemotherapy and radiation which would have left me with dentures, limited neck movement, vocal cord disability, and a possible lifetime feeding tube.

How did you change your diet and/or lifestyle following your cancer diagnosis? At whose suggestion?

With my own knowledge, I immediately began juicing and eating a more raw diet. After reading about Dr. Kerry's enzyme protocol for curing cancer, I put myself on an extensive enzyme program. I also received ozone treatments twice a week. I knew it was important to detox and gave myself coffee enemas.

After seven months on this therapy, I had a PET scan which indicated the cancer had spread. Then with the financial help of my church and a community fundraiser, I found an oncologist in Tijuana, Mexico, who treated my cancer with IV treatments of vitamin C, Laetrile, and minimal chemotherapy and cobalt radiation. (This type of radiation is outlawed in the USA.) I was cured as a result of my treatment in Mexico.

What treatment/lifestyle modification do you feel worked best for you? And why?

My oncologist referred me to a biological dentist who I believe found the major cause of my cancer—two teeth with root canals that were long-term infected and which the dentist extracted. I believe my highly knowledgeable, compassionate, caring dentist saved my life! I never knew the extensive dental connection to cancer and so many other degenerative diseases. He has enlightened me and so many others to the dangers of amalgam fillings, cavitations, and poor dental health. His website is www.mercury-free-dentist.com and his email is erichwolley@aol.com. I am thankful for my oncologist who eradicated my cancer, but I believe that without dental intervention, the cancer would have returned.

What treatment(s) do you continue to follow?

I drink a high-protein/super-green food shake and Essiac tea daily, take enzymes, colloidal minerals, vitamins B12, D, and C, cod liver oil, ubiquinol, and turmeric. A complete list of supplements and my sources can be found on my Caring Bridge website (login required) at www.debbiewylie.com.

What do you wish you had known when you were diagnosed? What advice do you have for someone receiving a cancer diagnosis today?

My advice would be to have a dentist remove and replace all your mercury fillings, root canals, and cavitations *safely* and put you on a lifetime health plan.

Detox, eat *clean* organic unprocessed foods, exercise, and forgive others!

What did you learn from having cancer?

I learned good health cannot be taken for granted. We need to research and find the *truth*. Our grocery shelves are full of over-processed foods, and our government allows toxic chemicals in our food that most other countries do not allow. We have to be *wise*. We are a *sick* country, full of food, but we are starving to death. In addition to our food crisis, our country is filled with legal drug pushers who are killing us!

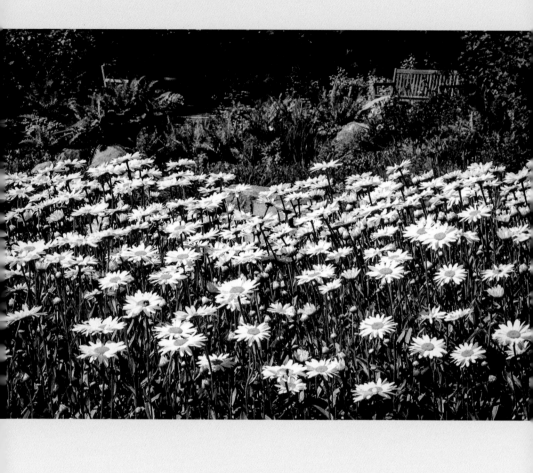

6

Hell No to Chemo

NOT EVERYONE WHO'S offered a chemo cocktail accepts that offer. Listening to their intuition, these women chose not to include chemo as a part of their treatment plan. Each one of them continues to believe they made the right choice.

Julia Chiappetta was living a fast-paced life when she was diagnosed with breast cancer. She knew intuitively that chemo was not for her. With the help of a friend, she began researching treatment options that were available to her and immediately transformed her diet and lifestyle. She became a strong advocate for herself and is now an equally strong advocate for other cancer patients. She volunteers for the annual Annie Appleseed Complementary and Alternative Medicine Conference, where she facilitates a cancer survivor panel each year that provides hope, inspiration, and valuable information for cancer patients.

Because of her sensitivity to chemicals, **Ann E. Fonfa** chose not to include chemo and radiation as a part of her treatment plan. Following surgery, she researched complementary and alternative treatments that would help to heal her cancer. With her husband supporting her every step of the way, Ann has become a passionate advocate for cancer patients. She travels the world to investigate treatment options and share her experiences. She also hosts a website (www.annieappleseedproject.org) that provides information for cancer patients and their families to assist them in navigating cancer care options. Ann also provides an invaluable service by hosting an annual conference connecting cancer patients and medical practitioners. Through this conference, cancer patients can access information about evidence-based complementary and alternative medicine.

Ruth Heidrich, Ph.D. saw an ad looking for people to be part of a clinical trial to study the relationship between diet and breast cancer. She jumped at this opportunity in 1993 and declined chemo and radiation. Dr. Ruth has been following a plant-based vegan diet ever since and is a vocal spokesperson sharing the benefits of healthy eating. Exercise is also an integral part of Dr. Ruth's life—she's an inspiring runner and dispels some long-held beliefs and myths about running in her book, *Lifelong Running*.

Melyssa Lawson was a young mother of two boys when she was diagnosed with cancer. A powerhouse with strong conviction, she listened to her inner voice and refused traditional treatment for thyroid cancer. She found a doctor who worked with her to put together an individualized treatment plan to heal her cancer. And now this mother of two is a mother of three—something her doctors told her would never happen. Never say never!

Diane Spilman-Giuliani believes her decision not to have chemo was the most important decision she made. She believes that building up her immune system with diet and lifestyle changes was exactly what her body needed. Cancer became a life-changing experience for Diane, as she used her time as a cancer patient to figure out what she was meant to do with her life. She became a health coach and helps people enjoy healthy living.

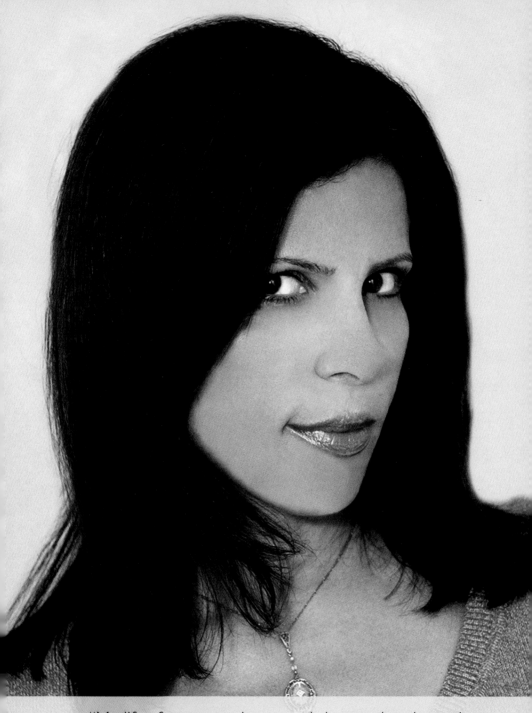

"My life after cancer is so much better than it used to be. I work fifty hours a week instead of ninety, and I'm able to support the cancer community."

Diagnosis: Stage IIb breast cancer (infiltrated ductal carcinoma)
Treatment: Lumpectomy, raw organic diet, juicing, focus on spirituality, fitness

What was the most important question you asked following your cancer diagnosis?

No one particular question comes to mind. I would say the most important thing I did was to become a strong advocate for myself. When I discovered a lump in my breast, the radiologist told me it was no problem. I just knew something was not right; I had to *demand* a biopsy.

Then doctors told me that I would die unless I had a double mastectomy, chemo, and radiation. Again, I had to listen to my inner voice. Before I could consider these drastic steps, I needed to learn about cancer and cancer treatment. I took two months off from work to read books, watch movies, listen to lectures, and interview doctors to realize I could heal my cancer with a completely natural protocol.

How did you change your diet and/or lifestyle following your cancer diagnosis? At whose suggestion?

A friend of mine is a scientist with a medical background; he volunteered to help me research treatment options. He went online every day for three months to help me identify the best treatment options for me.

My completely natural treatment included changes to my diet and lifestyle.

I got a dumpster and cleaned out my entire house—cleaning products, food, makeup, and microwave. I started by implementing a raw, organic diet. I was already physically active, and continued to include exercise as part of my treatment plan:

Raw organic diet	Antioxidants	Hydration
Rest	Fitness	Juicing
Enzymes	Spirituality	Education

Greens, seeds, nuts, quinoa, and wheatgrass shots became part of my daily healing regimen.

I also reduced my stress level by adjusting my work life and my extreme athleticism.

What treatment/lifestyle modification do you feel worked best for you? And why?

All of these elements were equally important to my healing. They provided a balance to my life that allowed me to regain my health. Wheatgrass was the key to my healing platform. Fourteen years later, I continue to follow this protocol—adjusted to reflect my current health—and share my experience with others whenever I can. I go to a clinic every year to check in on my health; based on my bloodwork, I tweak my supplementation plan and all of the other elements of my health plan.

What advice do you have for someone receiving a cancer diagnosis today?

Take an active role in creating your healing protocol because you've got to follow it for the rest of your life.

You need to have a sense of peace around the treatment path you select; it has to feel right for you.

There is no one magic bullet that will get you well; let your team of experts help you get well.

What did you learn from having cancer?

I learned to keep asking questions, and to trust my inner voice. This has led me to share my journey to health with men and women facing cancer diagnoses. I wrote a reference guide, *Breast Cancer—the notebook* (www.juliachiappetta.com/the-book.php), to help those who are newly diagnosed or those wishing to take a preventative approach toward health and wellness.

When I was researching cancer treatment, I came across the Annie Appleseed Project website. I found this site so helpful that I now help plan its annual conference.

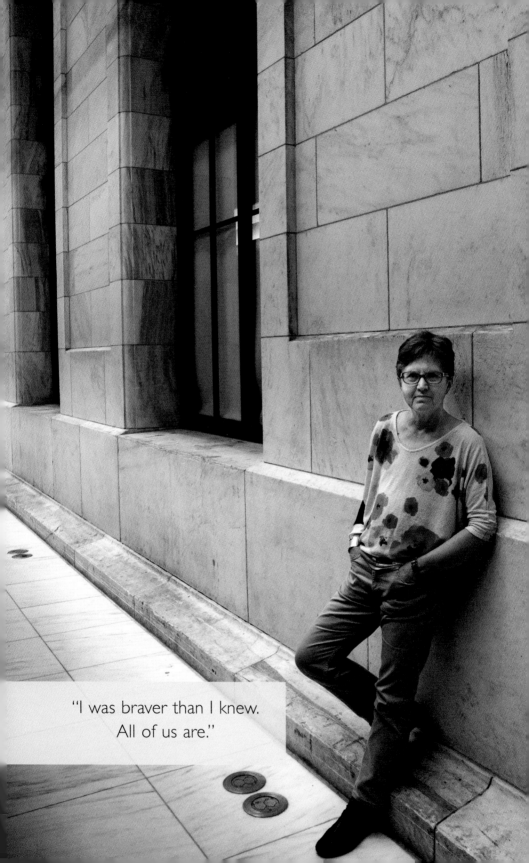

"I was braver than I knew.
All of us are."

Diagnosis: Stage I breast cancer (invasive lobular carcinoma)

Tell us about your diagnosis and treatment:

I was diagnosed with Stage I breast cancer in 1993. I had a lumpectomy, during which the doctor also removed several lymph nodes without my consent. This resulted in lymphedema—a permanent swelling of the arm—which continues to affect me on a daily basis.

Because I have multiple chemical sensitivities, I decided that chemotherapy wouldn't be good for me, nor radiation, and after surgery, made use of only alternative medicine.

Less than two years after my diagnosis, I had my first recurrence. In total since my original diagnosis, I've had twenty-five tumors—nine in the breast and fourteen on the chest wall. This led me to have three lumpectomies, two mastectomies and some random lump removals from the chest wall.

My complementary and alternative therapies have included:

Metabolic enzyme therapy	Applied kinesiology	714X (1 month instead of recommended 3)
Organic diet	Urine therapy	
Exercise	Supplements	Maitake mushroom D-fraction
Enjoyment	Chinese herbs	
Magnetic therapy	Gerson therapy	
	High-dose vitamin A	

I am very grateful to my husband, as he steadily supported me while all the docs offered was their viewpoint. While each successive tumor grew slower than normal cells, none of the doctors stepped up to say I was on the right track. Support groups have also been an important element of my treatment. I joined a support group in New York in 1993, and found that I wasn't the only one interested in exploring alternative therapies. This was the catalyst for establishing The Annie Appleseed Project in 1997—a volunteer-driven nonprofit organization that informs, educates, advocates and raises awareness around complementary and alternative medicine.

What treatment(s) do you continue to follow?

There are five things I do for my well-being every day to help reduce pollutant and toxic buildup in my body:

I eat real food—fresh (organic) fruits/vegetables—every day. I never eat junk food (no fried foods or soda) and I reduced salt, using herbs instead. I take dietary supplements that boost vitamins and nutrients good for my immune system.

I drink clean water.

I exercise moderately every day.

I apply detoxification methods that I have researched.

I do at least one thing every day that makes me happy and that relaxes me.

What do you wish you had known when you were diagnosed?

I wish I knew more about traditional Chinese medicine and the power of the herbs. I also wish I had known more about homeopathy.

What advice do you have for someone receiving a cancer diagnosis today?

Get involved with a support group.

Ask questions.

Let your friends and family help by caring for you, your home and your family. They want to.

There is no downside to eating healthy, exercising, detoxifying, and relaxing.

Stand up for what you believe in and in what works for you. If you are interested in complementary and integrative medicine, explore the studies to help you learn more so that you can decide what is best for you.

Visit my website, www.annieappleseedproject.org, which provides resources for cancer patients and their families. We host an annual education conference complete with organic food.

What else would you like to share?

I am not a doctor, I do not claim to be one. While I do not have medical training, I have spent more than twenty years attending medical conferences and gathering useful information. I am a Project LEAD, Food as Medicine and CancerGuides graduate. I am a patient. I am an advocate and an activist. I am driven to help others since I am now a twenty-plus-year survivor of breast cancer who never had chemotherapy (wasn't able to) nor radiation (declined) nor hormonal treatments (declined). Since I survived and have plenty of energy, I delight in helping others deal with the toxicity issues that conventional therapy brings or showing them options when that treatment fails to cure.

Ann E. Fonfa is the founder of Annie Appleseed Project: www.annieappleseedproject.org | www.facebook.com/annieappleseedproject

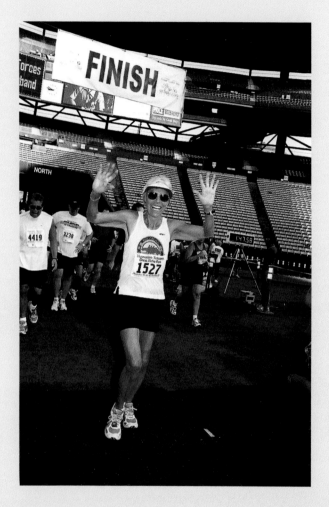

"I got a whole new education about the body and how it works in both health and disease. Most cancers are failures of the immune system to detect and destroy aberrant cells, and the Standard American Diet creates much disease and impairs the immune system. A low-fat vegan diet allows the immune system to do its job."

Diagnosis: Stage IV breast cancer

Treatment: When she was diagnosed at age forty-seven in 1982, Ruth began treatment with excisional biopsy (lumpectomy), followed by a modified radical mastectomy. She started a low-fat vegan diet two weeks later, despite her oncologist telling her that diet had nothing to do with breast cancer!

What was the most important question you asked following your cancer diagnosis?

What do we do now and what is my prognosis?

How did you change your diet and/or lifestyle following your cancer diagnosis?

Dr. John McDougall was looking for subjects for his clinical research trial to determine the role of diet in breast cancer. After speaking to him about the research available at that time, I elected to go with that as the only follow-on treatment after the surgery. *This meant no chemotherapy, radiation or hormonal manipulation: the only treatment variable was to be the low-fat vegan diet.*

I also intuitively knew that exercise was an important component of a healthy lifestyle. Since I was already a marathoner (a fourteen-year history as a daily runner), I decided to add swimming and cycling and to do the first of six Ironman triathlons and several ultra-marathons.

What treatment/lifestyle modification do you feel worked best for you? And why?

The primary modification was the low-fat vegan diet, and secondarily, my triathlon training, for a number of reasons. First, the symptoms regressed almost immediately. The excruciating bone pain subsided, the "hot spots" on the bone scans faded, the liver enzymes normalized, and the lesion in my lung encapsulated. I found I had more energy to not only continue the daily running but to add the swimming and cycling. I was able to sleep more soundly despite the anxiety and stress created by the cancer diagnosis. I almost immediately became optimistic about my prognosis.

What treatment(s) do you continue to follow?

Both the low-fat vegan diet and running, cycling, swimming with added weight training.

What advice do you have for someone receiving a cancer diagnosis today?

The standard medical protocol for cancer treatment is still chemotherapy and radiation after surgery, and I doubtless would have gone down that path except for the coincidence of finding that newspaper item looking for subjects for Dr. McDougall's research.

Obviously, I would advise everyone to follow a low-fat vegan diet and get lots of exercise. I still have hopes that the medical protocol will eventually catch up.

What else would you like to share?

Looking back over the past thirty years, it seems that what I did was so simple, although I realize that at the onset, it is scary and confusing because of a serious lack of medical and societal support to make these changes. Dr. McDougall recognized this as well and encouraged me to detail my journey from cancer to the Ironman in my book, *A Race for Life*. My website, www.ruthheidrich.com also has more details on how to do this.

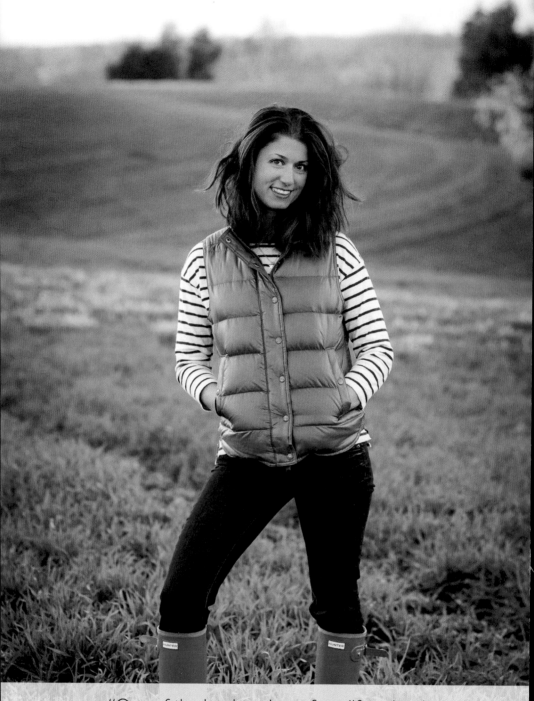

"One of the lousiest days of my life—the day
I heard I had cancer—allowed me to find the
life I was meant to live."

Melyssa Lawson

Diagnosis: Stage III papillary thyroid cancer
Treatment: Diet and lifestyle changes, no chemo or radiation

What was the most important question you asked following your cancer diagnosis?

What's my life expectancy? My doctor told me I would die if I didn't have surgery and radiation. I looked at people who were having surgery and radiation; they weren't doing well. I chose to walk down another path.

How did you change your diet and/or lifestyle following your cancer diagnosis? At whose suggestion?

My father connected me with a natural doctor. I followed a yeast-free diet, took supplements and began practicing yoga. I've always been a workout junkie and found that yoga kept me centered. After adapting to a yeast-free lifestyle, I juiced like a maniac, as many as four big juices a day. I alternated between colored and green juices, and even grew wheatgrass. I also incorporated Chinese herbs into my life two years after my diagnosis. I released stressful things from my life. And yes, that meant that some people who were in my life then no longer are today. I focus on relationships that deserve my energy and stay away from drama.

What treatment(s) do you continue to follow?

I continue to follow a plant-based diet—all organic—and check with my doctor to see if I need to take/adjust supplements. Yoga has become a way of life for me. I let the little things roll right off my back and try not to use unnecessary energy worrying about things that are out of my control. I still juice as well, but only twice a day.

What do you wish you had known when you were diagnosed?

I wish I knew the role that emotions would play in my recovery from cancer. I found that changing up my diet was fairly easy; the tough part for me was dealing with people. I discovered that some of my friendships weren't as solid as I thought they were. Because I didn't go through chemo and radiation, I looked healthy throughout my cancer treatment. While that's great, it also meant that some friends thought that meant I didn't need their support.

I also learned to make time for the people in my life who are important to me.

What advice do you have for someone receiving a cancer diagnosis today?

Don't be afraid.

Don't rush into any treatment. Take time to do some research, and weigh all your options.

Don't be bullied into following a treatment plan you're not comfortable with; listen to your instincts and stick to your convictions.

Don't look at your diagnosis as a death sentence: it's the first chapter to a whole new life.

What did you learn from having cancer?

I learned who I was and how to live fearlessly.

Anything you can dream or think—go for it!

I changed my thought process: I no longer say, I wish I could do this. Now I say, I'm going to make this happen!

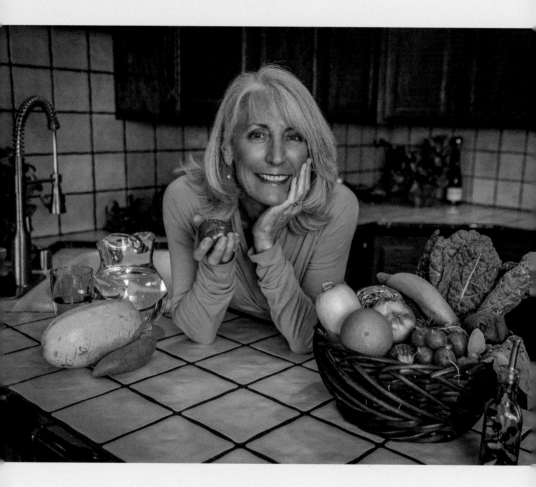

"Don't underestimate the healing power
of your food choices."

Diagnosis: Stage II breast cancer
Treatment: Lumpectomy followed by seven weeks of radiation therapy.

What was the most important question you asked following your cancer diagnosis?

Is chemotherapy absolutely necessary as part of my treatment plan?

How did you change your diet and/or lifestyle following your cancer diagnosis? At whose suggestion?

Initially I eliminated all refined sugars and high-glycemic foods and I increased my daily vegetable consumption.

A few months later, and after many hours of reading, I decided to switch to a plant-based diet. Today I eat a very small amount of animal protein (less than 5% of my diet). This includes cold-water wild-caught fish, 100% grass-fed beef, and free-range, hormone- and antibiotic-free poultry. Dairy makes up less than 3% of my diet.

My daily diet consists of a variety of vegetables and leafy greens, beans and legumes, and a wide variety of grains and grain-like seeds, and nuts. I limit my fruit to no more than two to three servings per day (sometimes less), and I eat mostly berries and citrus but include other fruits seasonally. I attempt to eat something green with every meal, and I like to include cruciferous vegetables as frequently as possible.

The suggestion to change to a plant-based diet came from T. Colin Campbell and Kris Carr.

What treatment/lifestyle modification do you feel worked best for you? And why?

I think choosing to *not* do any chemotherapy treatment was the best decision I could have made. I wanted to boost my immune system, not tear it down. I also feel that moving to a plant-based diet was a really wise lifestyle choice for me, too. I'm an A+ blood type and this diet works really well for me.

What treatment(s) do you continue to follow?

Because my breast cancer was estrogen receptor-positive, I was prescribed an aromatase inhibitor that I take daily.

What do you wish you had known when you were diagnosed?

I wish I had been more educated about the benefits of a plant-based diet. I grew up with a mostly meat-and-potatoes kind of diet and as a result, I fed my family similarly.

What did you learn from having cancer?

I learned to eat "Plant Strong" and to be more accepting and tolerant of myself and others, as well as to let go of the little things in life that are out of my control. I learned to love the gifts (good and not so good) that each day brings and how important my friends and loved ones are to me.

What else would you like to share?

When I was diagnosed with cancer, I was at a place in my life where I was beginning to question the purpose of the second half of my life. I had been searching for some way in which to serve my community in a bigger way and be personally fulfilled at the same time. Boom . . . I received my cancer diagnosis!

It was through my own journey of exploring what it means to have cancer and what else I could do about it, that I landed on what my "bigger purpose" was. It was only three months after my diagnosis that I decided to pursue a certification in health coaching so that I could guide others who were asking big questions such as, "What do I do *now?*"

Diane is now a nutrition and wellness educator with Wellness Within: www.wellnesswithin.org.

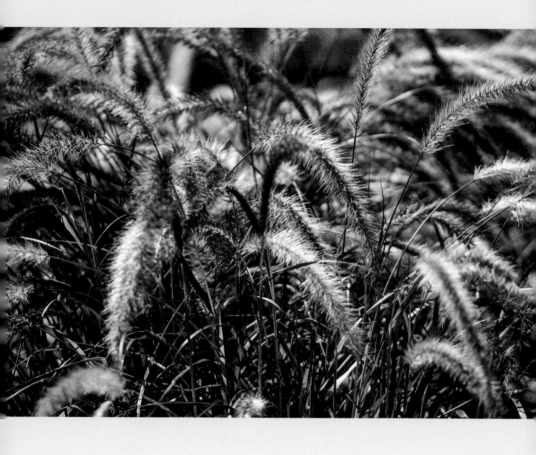

7

The Power of Prevention

L EARNING THE STORIES of all these brave cancer conquerors makes me ask, what if? What if there were a way to avoid being diagnosed in the first place? Well, maybe there is. And, certainly, the story of **Ellen Jaffe Jones** does not prove that a healthy diet and strong exercise program will keep you cancer-free. We've seen throughout this book the instances where people also reduced their stress, turned to friends and family for support, and explored their spirituality upon being diagnosed with cancer. Many, many factors influence whether cancer cells will overpower your immune system.

I've included Ellen's story here as a powerful example of how she overcame some health issues with diet and lifestyle choices. She's also managed to keep cancer at bay while many of her family members who followed different diet and lifestyle choices were prone to cancer diagnoses.

A staunch advocate for the vegan lifestyle, Ellen inspires and motivates her many followers to make conscious decisions—decisions that will support, rather than weaken, their immune system;

decisions that will nourish both their body and their soul; decisions that will support sustainable living.

A visit to her website (www.vegcoach.com) shows that this commitment to healthy living suits Ellen well: "As of May 2018, she has placed in 136 5K or longer races since 2006 'just' on plants. She has competed and placed nationally in multiple events in the National Senior Games. She is currently ranked 3rd in the USW65-69 4x100 meters, 5th in the 800 meters and 7th in the 1500 and 400 meters. She's done 2 marathons and 12 half marathons since 2011, something most sprinters with her speed don't ever do."

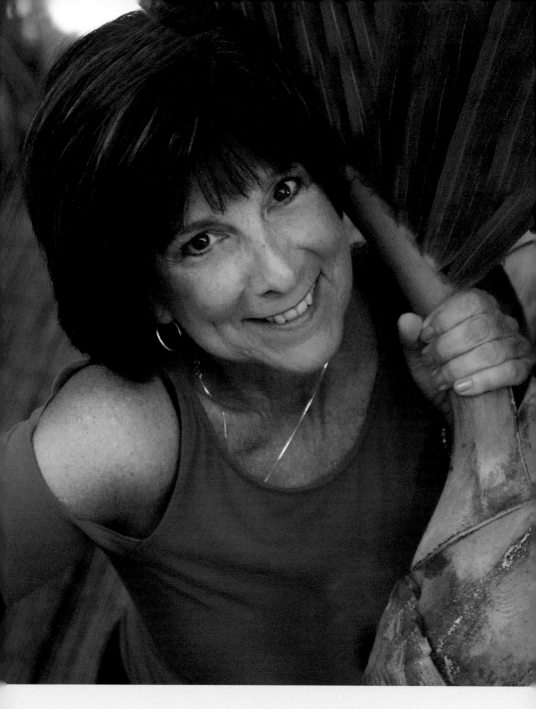

"While I don't have any way to prove it,
I believe that my healthy lifestyle has kept
cancer out of my life."

Is there a history of cancer in your family?

There's a long history of cancer in my family. My mother, aunt, and both sisters had breast cancer. Poor health in my family doesn't stop at cancer: my parents and all four of my grandparents had heart disease as well as diabetes.

Why did you change your diet to protect your health?

There have been two occasions in my life where I changed my diet to protect my health. First, when I was twenty-eight I was hospitalized with a severe colon blockage. Doctors told me I could avoid surgery if I changed my diet. I found a diet change much more appealing than surgery, so I immediately read every book I could get my hands on and decided to follow a mostly plant-based macrobiotic diet for a year. As my work became more stressful, I discovered the McDougall Plan (low-fat, vegan diet) was a better fit for my lifestyle.

Over the years, after my children were born and I re-entered the workforce, I gradually relaxed my nutrition standards until I found I was not eating a healthy diet. My body sent me a second message loud and clear that I needed to do something when I landed in the hospital with hemorrhaging fibroid tumors. Doctors in the emergency room recommended removal of the non-cancerous fibroids, as well as a hysterectomy. Fortunately, I called my doctor, who put the brakes on having surgery.

My doctor reminded me that I had had no health issues while following a low-fat, plant-based diet. She suggested I give that a try for three weeks. I followed her advice, and haven't looked back—and that was in 2004.

How has changing your diet impacted your health?

The numbers seem to tell it all—my cholesterol levels and weight both increased as I added dairy, meat, and processed foods into my diet; those numbers also decreased as I removed dairy, meat, and processed foods from my diet.

The real payoff for me, though, is that I feel so much better when I follow a low-fat, plant-based diet. As I lost weight, my energy level soared and I began running on a regular basis. Time flies. In my mid-60's now, I continue to run ten to thirty miles a week depending on my upcoming race. In 2017, I am a ranked sprinter—nationally and in Florida. Rare for someone with my sprint times, I have also finished two marathons and six half-marathons, placing in my age group in one of those.

What did you do to educate yourself about plant-based eating?

I knew I had to find a way to stay healthy. The skills from my eighteen-year career in journalism translated nicely for me in researching nutrition and health. I saw the positive relationship surrounding eating a plant-based diet, exercise, and health.

I decided to take the training offered by the Physicians Committee for Responsible Medicine and now teach cooking classes at hospitals, community centers, health food stores, and condo associations. I also became a certified personal trainer and running coach.

Do you feel that your lifestyle has kept you from having cancer?

It seems to me that the cancer diagnoses and other chronic diseases that have affected my family are a result of lifestyle rather than genetics. I work hard every day to stay healthy, and I feel better at sixty-two than I have at any other time in my life.

What suggestions do you have for people who are making changes to their diet and lifestyle?

While some people do best deciding to change all at once on one day, others do better taking baby steps and going gradually. I wrote *Kitchen Divided* focused in part, on managing my life with my former non-vegan ex-husband.

Just because you transition using some of the many diverse faux meats doesn't mean you are destined to a life of processed foods, as some people fear. I'm all about asking, "What did Mother Nature intend? What did our ancestors really eat?" Enjoy foods in all colors of the rainbow and trust some of the hero vegan doctors and their websites who have been treating their patients successfully for decades. Follow the money and ask, "Who paid for the research? Who stands to gain financially?" and the answers will become clear.

What else would you like to share?

Following a low-fat, vegan diet has been a life-changing experience for me. I've gone from being a journalist to becoming an author; a fitness, health and vegan food coach/consultant (www.vegcoach.com and www.facebook.com/ellenjaffejones); and a certified personal trainer and running coach. Who knew? I'm so glad I paid attention to that wake-up call my fibroid tumors presented. I could not be any happier or healthier than I am today!

Afterword

Thank you for taking the time to read the stories shared in this book. I'd like to give you a bit more information about two of the people whose stories you just read: Joyce Foley and Carroll Tiernan. Both of these women have passed away, less than a year from the publication date of this book. I kept their stories in the book because they epitomize the title of this book: *Finding Health After Cancer*. Joyce and Carroll lived their lives to the fullest, with joy and grace. They both found health after cancer, though not for as long as we would have liked.

Each person who shared their story in this book found and forged a path to heath that suited him or her best. I hope you've found inspiration from these stories. Stay curious: ask questions, take action, become an advocate – for yourself or friends and family who need someone to help them maneuver through, or avoid, a cancer diagnosis.

On the following pages you'll find a list of Resources: books I've read and websites I've visited to help me formulate questions, find answers, and stay engaged with the health care community. Pick up a book or two, visit a website or two, and see what information resonates with you as you explore health care options.

There are differing viewpoints in these books and websites. One point, however, seems clear to me: we are in control of our health care choices and must be informed consumers.

Resources

Books

The End of Illness by David B. Agus, MD

Cancer: 50 Essential Things to Do by Greg Anderson

Wake Up! You're Alive, But Are You Living? by Allison Andrews

The Whole-Food Guide for Breast Cancer Survivors by Edward Bauman, MEd, PhD and Helayne Waldman, MS, EdD

Life Over Cancer by Keith I. Block, MD

How We Do Harm by Otis Webb Brawley, MD, with Paul Goldberg

Thrive by Brendan Brazier

Thrive Foods by Brendan Brazier

The Blue Zones, Second Edition: 9 Lessons for Living Longer from the People Who've Lived the Longest by Dan Buettner

The China Study by T. Colin Campbell, PhD with Thomas M. Campbell II

32 Ways to Outsmart Cancer: Create a Body in Which Cancer Cannot Thrive by Dr. Nalini Chilkov, L.Ac., O.M.D.

Living Foods for Optimum Health by Brian R. Clement with Theresa Foy DiGeronimo

The Living Foods Lifestyle by Brenda Cobb

A World Without Cancer by Margaret I. Cuomo, MD

Heal Breast Cancer Naturally by Dr. Veronique Desaulniers

Take Control of Your Cancer by James W. Forsythe, MD, HMD

Never Fear Cancer Again by Raymond Francis, MSc

Super Immunity by Joel Furman, MD

Being Mortal: Medicine and What Matters in the End by Atul Gawande

The Gerson Therapy by Charlotte Gerson and Morton Walker, DPM

There's No Place Like Hope by Vickie Girard

A Race for Life by Ruth Heidrich, Ph.D.

Lifelong Running by Ruth Heidrich, Ph.D.

Cancer-Free: Your Guide to Gentle, Non-Toxic Healing by Bill Henderson and Carlos M. Garcia, MD

Eat Vegan on $4 a Day: A Game Plan for the Budget-Conscious Cook by Ellen Jaffe Jones

Kitchen Divided: Vegan Dishes for Semi-Vegan Households by Ellen Jaffe Jones

Surviving After Cancer: Living the New Normal by Anne Katz

The Macrobiotic Way by Michio Kushi

Hope: 30 Tips to Overcome Cancer Naturally by Dr. Christine Maguire

The Cancer Killers: The Cause is the Cure by Dr. Charles Majors and Dr. Ben Lee with Sayer Ji

When Hope Never Dies by Marlene Marcello-McKenna

Little Changes by Kristi Marsh

A Survivor's Guide to Kicking Cancer's Ass by Dena Mendes

Unexpected Recoveries by Tom Monte

F**ck-Off Cancer by Linda Brossi Murphy

The Raw Life by Paul Nison

Food Over Medicine by Pamela Popper, PhD, ND and Glen Merzer

In Honor of Them: Life's Lessons from Cancer by Denise Morin

The Hip Chick's Guide to Macrobiotics by Jessica Porter

Keep it Simple, Keep it Whole: Your Guide to Optimum Health by Alona Pulde, MD and Matthew Lederman, MD

Beating Cancer with Nutrition by Patrick Quillin, PhD, RD, CNS

Kicking Cancer in the Kitchen by Annette Ramke and Kendall Scott

Mind Over Medicine by Lissa Rankin, MD

n of 1 by Glenn Sabin with Dawn Lemanne, MD, MPH

Mom's Marijuana by Dan Shapiro

Love, Medicine & Miracles by Bernie Siegel, MD

Your Child Doesn't Have to Die by Leanne Sorteberg with Lisa C. Ragsdale

Forks Over Knives: The Cookbook by Del Sroufe

The Perfect Formula Diet by Janice Stanger, PhD

Radical Remission: Surviving Cancer Against All Odds by Kelly A.
    Turner, PhD
Macrobiotics for Dummies by Verne Varona
Nature's Cancer-Fighting Foods by Verne Varona
The Great Life Diet by Denny Waxman
The Hippocrates Diet and Health Program by Ann Wigmore
A Life in the Balance by Meg Wolff
Becoming Whole by Meg Wolff with Tom Monte
Food Fix: Ancient Nourishment for Modern Hungers by Susan Lebel
    Young

Websites

Annie Appleseed Project ~ www.annieappleseedproject.org and
    www.facebook.com/annieappleseedproject
Block Center Integrative Cancer Treatment ~ www.blockmd.com
Julia Chiappetta ~ www.juliachiappetta.com
Cancer Decisions ~ cancerdecisions.com
Cancer Treatment Centers of America ~ www.cancercenter.com
Chris Beat Cancer ~ www.chrisbeatcancer.com
T. Colin Campbell Center for Nutrition Studies ~
    www.facebook.com/nutritionstudies
Christina Cooks ~ www.christinacooks.com
Dena's Healthy U ~ www.denashealthyu.com
Elizabeth's Gone Raw ~ elizabethsgoneraw.com
Family Chiropractic Associates ~ scarboroughfamilychiro.com
Green Med Info ~ www.greenmedinfo.com
Dr. Michael Greger nutritionfacts.org and www.drgreger.org
Harmony Haven Healing Arts ~ www.harmonyhavenhealingarts.com
Hand-Crafted Health ~ www.handcrafted-health.com
Ruth Heidrich, Ph.D. ~ www.ruthheidrich.com
Hippocrates Health Institute ~ hippocratesinst.org
Kris Carr ~ kriscarr.com
The Kicking Kitchen ~ thekickingkitchen.com
Less Cancer | Prevention is the Future ~ www.lesscancer.org

Living Foods Institute ~ www.livingfoodsinstitute.com

Dr. MacDougall's Health & Medical Center ~ www.drmcdougall.com

Macro Vegan / Marlene Watson-Tara ~ macrovegan.org and
     marlenewatsontara.com

The Organic Coach® ~ www.theorganiccoach.com

Physicians Committee for Responsible Medicine ~ www.pcrm.org

Dr. Pam Popper ~ drpampopper.com

Purple Iris Foundation / Christina Parrish ~
     www.purpleirisfoundation.com

The Real Truth About Health ~ www.therealtruthabouthealth.com

Strengthening Health Institute ~ shimacrobiotics.org

Stupid Cancer ~ stupidcancer.org

Thankful Foods ~ www.thankfulfoods.com

The Truth About Cancer ~ thetruthaboutcancer.com

The Veg Coach ~ www.vegcoach.com and
     www.facebook.com/ellenjaffejones

Wealth Thru Nutrition, "The Nutritional Epigenics Company" ~
     www.wealththrunutrition.com

Wellness Forum Health ~ wellnessforumhealth.com

Wellness Within ~ www.wellnesswithin.org

Whole Health Acupuncture and Herbal Medicine ~
     www.acupunctureinmaine.com

Debbie Wylie ~ www.debbiewylie.com

Your Own Wellness ~ www.arpnaturod.com

About the Author

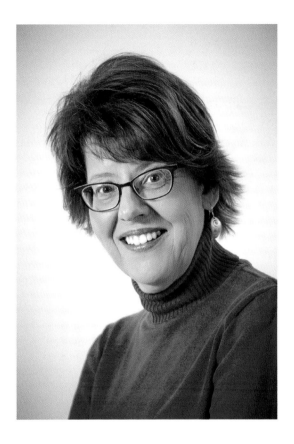

While curiosity may have killed the cat, being curious and asking questions keeps Deb going every day. When she came across the phrase below, Deb folded the page over and found herself returning to it over and over again – each time, she asked a new question: What does that mean? Why is there no footnote? Why had she never heard this before?

"It is impossible for cancer to develop in an alkaline environment." (This seemingly simple phrase appears in Brendan Brazier's book *Thrive: The Vegan Nutrition Guide to Optimal Performance in Sports and Life.*)

The more Deb read, the more she realized that each one of us can take control of our health. She read of people overcoming health obstacles when history indicated that wasn't possible. She learned of people becoming strong health advocates for themselves and others. And she wanted to learn more.

So began a wild and wonderful journey as Deb talked with people, attended conferences and workshops, and kept on reading. All of this brought her to changing her own life: while researching and writing this book, she enrolled in a program at the Institute for Integrative Nutrition. She is now an Integrative Nutrition Health Coach, working with people to help them achieve their health goals.

Stay curious. Ask questions. Take control of your health.